YOU REALLY DON'T HAVE TO!

Natural Therapy Updated

by
Herald Maleske, M.Div., Ph.D.

The Natural Therapy Foundation Press
Irvine, California

Copyright © 1980
by
HERALD MALESKE, M.Div., Ph.D.

Cloth: ISBN 0-937792-00-4
Library of Congress Catalog No. 80-52427

First Edition
1980

Printed in the United States of America

The Natural Therapy Foundation Press
5 Greenleaf
Irvine, California 92714

2288111

to "Gussie,"
my sainted mother,
who lived her long life
according to the healing principles
described in the pages that follow . . .

CONTENTS

foreword . . . Hans Selye, M.D., Ph.D., D.Sc.

by way of introduction . . . h.m.

chapter   **page**

Nature,
to be commanded,
must be obeyed.
    —Francis Bacon

foreword ...

I am pleased to have been asked to write a foreword to *You Don't Really Have To!* by Dr. Herald Maleske. Having reviewed his first book *Natural Therapy,* I realized Dr. Maleske to be a man who not only could state the case of a particular therapy clearly, but who also had an obvious love for the process and for his community.

Response to the subject of Natural Therapy was great enough to encourage Dr. Maleske to update the first volume. This favorable response does not surprise me; in my travels throughout the world to discuss my own particular interest—the field of stress—I am constantly confronted by people who are seeking ways to reduce the distress of modern life.

Although I have not done any specific research on Natural Therapy and cannot claim any expertise in this field, I fully support any treatment that helps us cope with the unpleasant effects of stress. I have had an opportunity to discuss emotional and behavioral problems with many health practitioners, and seeing this volume, which brings together the findings of several important researchers, leads me to conclude that there must indeed be something illuminating in Natural Therapy, something that certainly merits further attention and research.

When I first encountered stress as the "syndrome of just being sick" in 1936, I gave little thought to its psychological or sociological implications, for I saw stress as a purely physiological, chemical, and medical phenomenon. The growing interest in this field, however, evidenced by the tremendous response of the general public to some of my nontechnical books, made me realize that stress affects and therefore intrigues everyone, no matter what his education or profession.

There is a need, then, for books on all levels that explain how we can best minimize the distress of suffering and disease while maximizing the good stress or "eustress" of accomplishment and happiness. I have therefore developed a code of behavior which I call "altrusitic egoism," a set of guidelines that help us to live in harmony with our biological drives and aspirations.

But there are several approaches to better understanding and no set of guidelines can apply to each person in every situation. For many the general approach of *You Don't Really Have To!*, an application of psychological techniques within a Christian context—so closely related to the code of "altruistic egoism"—may be the most appealing. At all events, the two approaches do not compete but rather complement each other. Like my code, Natural Therapy focusses on human well-being, teaching us to reflect on our major goals for the survival and progress of humankind.

Hans Selye
President, International
Institute of Stress,
Montreal, Canada

by way of introduction ...

When Natural Therapy first came into being about five years ago, and first appeared in published form about two years after that, we never really doubted that it would survive, and we had even advertised is as "a new yet old therapy." Its form was new, but the principles upon which it is based are as old as natural law, and thus older than humankind itself. So we are not surprised to be writing another book about it.

What is a little amazing to us is that this book, which seeks to describe a therapy that, already in these few intervening years, has matured into a rather complete one, seems to us to be all too inadequate to present the far-reaching applications of it that are already possible, let alone the vast, and as yet unexplored, possibilities for it that, day in and day out, are brought to our attention.

With that kind of situation the reader can imagine the difficulty of trying to write a book, not too long, but still covering the subject, that is often desired these days. It has been correctly observed that, if a therapy can be put in a nutshell, that's where it really belongs, and we heartily agree.

At the same time, there are a lot of people out there that are hurting and could be helped by this therapy. So there is also an urgency to try to get the basic information to them as soon as possible.

To try to overcome these formidable obstacles of time and space, we were somehow led to present the information this book desires to impart in a manner that transgresses one of the basic and time-honored laws of successful writing — avoid having two basically different audiences in mind for the same book.

Too often the information falls into the cracks, and is useful for neither, or less useful to both. But, we thought, that might be generally true, and still Natural Therapy had something special going for it. Because it emphasized the natural, it's quite likely that there would be vast areas where the two audiences would overlap in natural knowledge and consequent interest.

Knowing full well another basic law about writing — that, if one cannot define one's audience, one does not have one — we felt confident that we knew well the two audiences we wanted to reach — therapists and those in need of therapy for significant problems. One cannot be a good therapist without also knowing a great deal about human beings and their problems. And one cannot be adequately helped in therapy without an adequate understanding of the therapeutic approach of the therapist.

And we had one more thing going for us in this approach. While it is true that the therapist is essentially professional, academic, and technical, and the client is rather amateur, practical, and not too technical in typical approaches to the area of human behavior, there are large areas of overlap. For one, if one of our mentors, psychiatrist Camilla Anderson, is right about members of her own profession, therapists are among the foremost of those who could, in their own typical kinds of problems, be helped by using our therapy. And, for another, this book, like its predecessor, was designed to present a self-help approach to problems; thus the one in need of therapy also acts in the role of a therapist.

The reader will soon note how this dual, yet overlapping approach, is carried out. Usually preliminary information is given, often in a more theoretical and/or technical vein, and this is usually followed, often without too much transition, by rather blunt and plain directions of a definite and practical nature. If both the reader who is a therapist by trade, and the reader who is mainly in need of therapy at this time, will always view the information given from both points of view, for which they also have a natural interest, our dual approach will actually prove to be more helpful.

Some readers may note that there is more than the usual

amount of repetition normally found in books of this kind. Many years of teaching members of wide age groups have amply demonstrated to us that the old observation that "repetition is the mother of studies" is still valid, so it is not just our long association with the U. S. Air Force that induces us also here to "tell 'em what you're gonna say, say it, then tell 'em what you said," as the military used to advise.

Actually, since individuals with significant problems are usually very impatient and tend to move too rapidly and with too little concentration, as the reader will soon understand, they often miss and misunderstand some of the essentials. Repetition, time and again, of such essentials is our way of trying to better equip them, for their upcoming battle, with all the weapons that they need as well as the complete knowledge of how to use them.

Just one final note. While we have some sympathy for the complaints of feminists, limitations of space make it necessary for us to use the terms that refer to males to include, where obvious, also females. Occasionally, however, we depart from that general practice, just to indicate our partial agreement with the complaint about it.

We've set the stage. Now it's your turn to perform.

h.m.

chapter **1**

*Natural Therapy
And The Cause of
Significant Problems*

THIS BOOK IS MAINLY ABOUT HAVE-TOS

In the realm of therapy a have-to is generally regarded as a compulsion or force within an individual that can compel that individual to act in ways that often produce significant problems in his life. The purpose of this present volume is to help individuals to both solve and prevent such problems by assisting them to recognize the presence of have-tos and to learn to control them. While there may also exist have-tos that appear to be constructive ones that produce only good, in our opinion the only good have-tos have more "want-to" about them than "have-to" and thus are not really have-tos at all. To understand more fully the part that have-tos play in problems it is important for you to know how we ourselves discovered them.

WE DISCOVERED HAVE-TOS WHEN
WE FASHIONED NATURAL THERAPY

Natural Therapy is the title of our first book about important human problems, and it was designed especially to be a self-help book for emotional and behavior problems. In this and the following chapter we hope to summarize the very first public presentation of Natural Therapy as it appeared in our first book about it. In that first attempt to present Natural Therapy we decided to include only the bare essentials, for we were mostly interested in obtaining some early feedback.

But now that we have received a sufficient amount of that, we present our original Natural Therapy in this second book in much greater detail, even though that is not the prime purpose of this volume, which is designed to *update* the therapy and make it much more helpful, now that it has been put to use in many differing situations. In addition to these improvements, which will be described later in this book, the additional detail that we are presenting in the first two chapters includes a description of how we were led to some of the components of this unique system of therapy. This will have the additional advantage of making it easier to understand and accept.

NATURAL THERAPY HAS A LONG HISTORY

While you may not have heard of Natural Therapy before, after you read this description of it you will realize that it is as old as humankind. It has always been around. That's one reason why we have called it *Natural* Therapy. For various reasons, however, humans have generally overlooked it. Apparently only a minority in every age have been aware of it and used it to their advantage. Others, though they did not really know about it, happened to use it, rather unconsciously, for their benefit. Still others, also using it quite unconsciously, erroneously credited their good fortune to other factors, sometimes even writing "success" books about them. But, when others try to use their formula for success, too, they, of course, fail to achieve the promised and the desired results. The reason is apparent.

INTUITIVELY WE ALL HAVE AN INKLING
ABOUT NATURAL THERAPY

While Natural Therapy has been generally overlooked by people, the experiences of life have the habit of bringing it, however faintly, to their attention. How often, for example, haven't you despised yourself when you realized that you had acted with great selfishness. How good you felt when you gave help to others. That was Natural Therapy trying to get its foot in the door.

Natural Therapy, as advocated by the writer of this book, had its beginning in the writer's life many years ago. In the early years of our pastoral ministry, we sometimes counseled individuals on the basis of principles which were not generally advocated in the current books on counseling, but which came to us rather intuitively out of the situation.

We recall very vividly the time one of our most faithful and attractive parishioners rushed into our office one day greatly disturbed. She had just come from a bake sale which our ladies were conducting, and she was upset because she was wondering what the ladies must think of her. She had brought only one cake to the sale, and all the ladies, she was sure, knew that she had both the time and the money to bring several cakes. These ladies surely must despise her for this. But she became upset even further when we gave this abrupt reply: "What makes you think that those ladies ever think twice about you at all?" We wish we could say that we followed this up with some additional Natural Therapy which would have helped her more to solve her problem, but at that time we were still greatly ignorant of all that was involved in Natural Therapy.

We cite this incident to show that in those early days we knew intuitively what was the cause of some problems that individuals experienced — their own grandiosity. We will describe shortly the part that grandiosity plays in human problems.

Before going on, however, let us relate another incident

from those earlier days which suggests that we knew intuitively also about other aspects of Natural Therapy. A married couple, who were not members of our congregation, came in for counseling one day. The wife had already had divorce papers served on her husband, but both were still a little in doubt about whether a divorce was the best answer to their problem. After we heard their story we told them that they were not living according to the rules of life, and that we could not help them unless they did. When they asked what the rules of life were, we proceeded to tell them, dwelling especially upon their need to be interested more in helping each other than in only helping themselves.

That advice, too, illustrated the heart of Natural Therapy, although we did not recognize its full import at the time. We might add that this couple followed that advice, and the divorce papers were torn up. We did not realize it fully then, but Natural Therapy really works.

NATURAL THERAPY DEVELOPED IN OUR EXPERIENCES

We wish we could state that those early inklings of Natural Therapy led to a rapid development of a complete therapy, but twenty-five more years had to pass before we realized that we should have paid more attention to what we intuitively felt about human behavior. Those were agonizing years in many respects, for, while we were still very much involved with people and their problems, we found we did not usually help them very much, especially with their emotional and behavior problems. John (we've changed the name) kept on going on his alcohol binges, embarrassing his very fine family. And Susan (we've changed her name, too) continued to experience terrifying emotional upsets to the point where she was beginning to doubt whether she did have a proper religious faith. This short list would not be complete without also mentioning the neighborhood "eccentric" who loudly kept telling everyone around how she got the Lutheran preacher to give her the "last rites" (even though she was not dying, and Lutherans do not believe in "last rites").

We now know why we usually failed to help them. We were constantly sidetracked by what psychologists and psychiatrists were usually advocating as the causes and the solutions of emotional and behavior problems. Some of what they claimed was true, but much of it was not true, and it failed to help for any length of time, especially in the more difficult problems. Of course it should also be stated that we turned to the behavioral scientists only after we found that the usually-advocated spiritual remedies of religion did not help very much either. We now know also why spiritual remedies usually fail. We deal with that problem at some length especially in a later chapter of this book.

At any rate we finally resigned our job and dropped everything else to concentrate on finding the solution to human problems. Our greatest interest was in emotional and behavior problems, for they were the most difficult as well as the most painful ones, and they played some part in every solution to any problem.

Researching a great deal of what has been written on the subject, it was inevitable that we should achieve some new insights into it. The writings of Alfred Adler, Hans Eysenck, and Camilla Anderson were most useful in acquiring those new insights. Some publications of Albert Ellis and a workshop conducted by him also confirmed some of the things that Adler, Eysenck, and Anderson were saying. These new insights, coupled with the knowledge and experiences we had acquired previously, formed the basis from which finally our Natural Therapy emerged.

If you have already read *Natural Therapy,* you also have a good foundation for gaining additional insights into Natural Therapy through the reading of this subsequent book, which is essentially a summary of what was in the first book, together with some very important newer discoveries about it which we have made as a result of our own and others' early experiences with Natural Therapy. Chapters one and two of this book present essentially the information in book one, but add so much more, by way of further explanation of it, that no one should skip the reading of them before going on to the others.

NATURAL THERAPY WAS ORIGINALY AIMED AT EMOTIONAL AND BEHAVIOR PROBLEMS

While every problem has emotional and behavioral aspects, there are some problems which are essentially emotional and some that are essentially behavioral. Examples of emotional problems are such common ones as undue anxiety, excessive fear, oppressive feelings of inferiority and inadequacy, an unshakable feeling of guilt, etc. Examples of behavior problems are continuing inability to get along with others, failure to observe important rules of behavior, delinquency, criminality, etc. Of course, we all have emotional and behavior problems of a sort at times, but usually they are only moderate ones and are more or less of short duration. The emotional and behavior problems in which we were interested were those that were chronic, acute, serious, and their causes were largely unknown to the one with the problem, and, for that reason, it was difficult to modify or eliminate them.

It was for such problems that Natural Therapy was originally fashioned. It was realized, of course, that such problems sometimes have physical or organic causes, and for that reason Natural Therapy has always advised that those with such problems first consult a competent physician. But, even if there is a physical cause, Natural Therapy can help the individual cope with his problems while medical treatment is being administered and as long as emotional or behavioral symptoms persist.

While most self-help books deal essentially with emotional problems, *Natural Therapy* deals also with behavior problems, for it was discovered that functional problems of emotion and behavior have essentially the same cause and consequently the same basic solution.

GRANDIOSITY WAS FOUND TO BE THE DIRECT CAUSE OF EMOTIONAL AND BEHAVIOR PROBLEMS

While there is no widespread agreement among psychologists, psychiatrists, and behavioral scientists in general about the causes of *behavior* problems, as is evidenced by the many and varied theories of the causes of crime and delinquency, there is general agreement that a common casuse of *emotional* problems is a feeling of inferiority. But, while Natural Therapy agrees that feelings of inferiority are commonly found in emotional problems, it contends that the basic cause of both emotional and behavior problems is grandiosity.

By the term grandiosity we mean an unrealistic feeling of superiority that an individual with significant emotional and behavior problems has acquired earlier. The individual that is grandiose feels more than the normal degree of self-regard found in the average person; he feels that he is someone extra-special, that he is not "common clay," that he is at least a notch or two above others and is entitled to be highly regarded and catered to by them, that things should be easy for him, that his value-system is best. Grandiosity is excessive false pride, often referred to as egotism or egocentricity.

Many psychologists and psychiatrists, while seeing inferiority as the common basic problem, often mention the obvious egocentricity of the person with *emotional* problems, but somehow they don't seem to know how to fit it in, and they seldom aim at it in their treatment of the individual. Some even see egocentricity in *behavior* problems, for there it is usually quite obvious, but they usually view it as an overcompensation for basic inferiority, and they aim their treatment at inferiority.

Of course, there have been a few therapists who have seen the part that grandiosity plays. Alfred Adler, an early defector from Freud, described the interplay between inferiority and superiority, but basically he tended to view superiority as overcompensation for inferiority, which it sometimes is, but that, too, he failed to see, is also motivated by frustrated grandiosity. Adler, however, made much of the superiority resulting from parental pampering as an important factor in emotional and behavior problems, but he did not explain why some pampered children have problems while others do not.

Karen Horney wrote about the so-called "idealized self-image" that emotionally disturbed individuals often display. This "idealized self-image" has all the characteristics of the grandiosity we have been describing. However, psychiatrist Horney did not describe this as a cause of the problem, but as something that apparently develops as a result of the problem.

Both Adler and Horney had the ingredients for fashioning a therapy that would really work. Both saw that superiority was highly visible in the midst of all the inferiority that apparently produced the problems. But they both made the same basic mistake. They failed to see that superiority was prior. For thirty years we had made the same mistake.

To Adler's credit it should be pointed out here that he devised a therapy that was aimed at eliminating superiority, but it was too weak to do the job that needs to be done to modify the kind of grandiosity that, Natural Therapy contends, is the real cause of problems.

While we had always suspected that something like grandiosity was inherent in emotional and behavior problems, it was not until we chanced to read an article by Camilla Anderson that we not only received some confirmation of our suspicions, but also were led to give serious attention to an idea floating around in our mind that, until then, seemed too impossible to be true — the idea that egocentricity was somehow the cause of all inferiority feelings.

We had tried for thirty years to help people with their inferiorities, which were produced, the professionals were always telling us, by earlier experiences, and all we were ending up with was a greater respect for the power of earlier experiences, for, when we attacked them in order to help people with problems, we could never seem to overcome their apparent influence. But, as time passed, we began to suspect that, no matter what the problem was, the real problem always seemed to be that the individual involved could not get himself off his hands. Somehow it always seemed that the sufferer could not remove himself from the situation enough to reduce its effect upon him. In the whole problem he seemed to be able to see only himself. The problem always seemed to surround him like a mirror, for no matter what aspect of the problem he looked at, he could see in it only a reflection of himself.

Many times the thought crossed our mind that this is the reason why so much of psychotherapy today is so ineffective. Using modern therapeutic techniques, the therapist usually leads the patient to think about himself even more than he already usually does, thus really aggravating the real problem, which is that the patient thinks only of himself, and can't get himself off his hands. No wonder that therapists themselves are increasingly admitting their failures.

So, you see, we were really ready for Anderson's idea that the cause of problems was really grandiosity. On top of that, Camilla Anderson was a very reputable therapist, having held many important positions, including that of chief psychiatrist at the California Institution for Women. It was extremely important to us that a professional with such credentials should confirm what we had begun to suspect about the cause of problems. In addition, with her wide experience she was able to furnish us a complete and beautiful description of grandiosity; samples of her incredible grasp of human grandiosity are found in her writings, some of which are listed in the reference section at the end of this book, and which she is permitting us to edit and include in a projected book of readings.

It is easy to understand that grandiosity should play a

leading role in producing *behavior* problems. After all, if an individual is grandiose he will want to have his way, regardless of what someone else or even the law desires or directs.

Charles Colson, former aide to President Nixon, blamed his unacceptable behavior on his "damnable pride and ego." It is easy, in the light of what we have been saying, to understand his assessment of the cause of his problem.

But it is difficult to understand the part that grandiosity plays in the production of *emotional* problems. We have had very few people deny that grandiosity could be behind *behavior* problems. They apparently accept this quite readily because unacceptable behavior is usually labeled as "bad," and grandiosity usually also has a "bad" connotation for many. When, however, we tell people that grandiosity is also behind *emotional* problems, they usually agree that this may be true for a small number of people, but not for the vast majorty. They apparently have this notion, because seldom are people with emotional problems considered "bad" just because they have such problems, and it just does not seem right to label them as grandiose.

In fact, it is usually true that individuals with emotional problems are usually very fine people. They usually are honest, reliable, intelligent, sympathetic and law-abiding. One psychiatrist some years ago even wrote a book whose theme was that you should be thankful if you had emotional problems, for it proved that you were a very fine person. It's been my experience, however, that the sufferer would gladly give up many of his fine qualities if he could only get rid of his problem. He need not give up his fine qualities. He needs only to use those same qualities differently, as we later indicate.

While it is hard to understand that grandiosity is behind all emotional problems, as we have indicated, it becomes easy to accept this truth when one understands how grandiosity operates. Grandiosity, especially in persons who develop emotional problems, almost always masquerades as inferiority, fear, guilt, undue modesty, and the like.

And this is how such paradoxical manifestations come about.

Unlike the non-grandiose person who does not take failure so seriously, the grandiose person is constantly on the alert to prevent any kind of failure on his part, so he fears failure in almost any situation. It is this that makes him feel inferior and inadequate, for he is aware that he could fail, and he considers any failure to be awful, terrible, and catastrophic. What makes matters worse for him is that, as we have indicated earlier, he is usually quite intelligent, and he can thus discern more possibilities for failure than the not-so-intelligent person. Knowing the many possibilities of failure and fearing them so much, he usually acts in a humble, apologetic, and self-effacing manner. In this way he is reducing the extent of his fall and cushioning it should it occur. He is thus constantly keeping the back door open for the escape he may have to make.

He also feels that he has to act perfectly to avoid any diminishing of his grandiosity, both in his own eyes and in the eyes of others. Because it is impossible to behave perfectly, sooner or later he will have guilt feelings. This is not normal guilt from failure to live up to a code of behavior; normal guilt seldom lasts very long. This is *neurotic* guilt which persists because he is not able to forgive himself. He says to himself, as it were: "How could I, such a wonderful person that I am, how could I have ever done such a thing? What will people think of me?" While he may not show it (in fact, he is careful to conceal it), he is constantly struggling to retain an image of himself as always best, perfect, superior, and entitled to the deference and cooperation of others.

While grandiosity may manifest itself in self-display and arrogant and pompous behavior (such behavior, as we shall see later, does not cause any real problems for an individual), more frequently by far it masquerades as humility and self-effacement, a sure indication that grandiosity is causing some real problems. Usually the individual with *emotional* problems cloaks his grandiosity with the appearance of humility; when he doesn't, which is rarely, he covers his fear of failure or of being imperfect by appearing to be proud. Often the individual with *behavior* problems shows his grandiosity by appearing to be what he actually is — arrogant; when he doesn't, he covers his exaggerated self-feelings by acting humble in order to deceive those whom he seeks to victimize. The inability to recognize grandiosity from the paradoxical forms it often assumes has led many counselors astray.

After absorbing what we have stated thus far about grandiosity, you must be wondering if it is really true that grandiosity is at the root of all emotional and behavior problems. Your doubts may result from questions like these: Why has it taken so long to make this discovery, and why do so few behavioral scientists today acknowledge it? Believe me, we asked ourselves those questions many times, and we had to have satisfactory answers for them before we could write our books about this discovery.

Camilla Anderson must have wrestled with such questions, too, for, while she constantly found that her therapy worked when it was aimed at the elimination of grandiosity, she could not understand why other therapists failed to respond favorably to her discovery of the role of grandiosity.

We finally found at least a plausible and partial answer to such questions, oddly enough, through something that Anderson wrote in a paper she once delivered to a group of pastors. In that presentation she pointed out that, among the things that psychiatrists and pastors had in common, a feeling of personal grandiosity was a frequent one. Now, she certainly knew herself and many other psychiatrists, so she should know. In addition, she had many experiences with pastors in her life, having even considered becoming a medical missionary earlier in her life, and lecturing at many pastoral conferences in her career as a psychiatrist.

We, too, in the ministry for over thirty years, know ourself and hundreds of other pastors. We also have become acquainted with many behavioral scientists in our secondary role as a student and a professor in the behavioral sciences. And we concur wholeheartedly with Anderson's observation about the presence of grandiosity among psychiatrists and pastors.

The point we are making is that those who are grandiose are usually the last ones to see grandiosity and admit it. And it is the very ones who need most to see it — the therapists and the ones with emotional and behavior problems — who are the least interested in seeing it and the least able to see it. Lay people without significant emotional and behavior problems have no need to see it and are not looking for it.

To us, what we have stated in the previous paragraph provided a sufficient explanation for the long delay in the discovery of the role of grandiosity and the reluctance of therapists to recognize it. Another, and perhaps more plausible reason, becomes apparent when we consider, then, how it ever became possible that this discovery should ever be made, if those, that needed most to make it, were so incapable of doing so.

As one who has taught courses in social change, we are well aware of the difficulty of assigning reasons for the making of an important discovery at a particular time in history. While social scientists often cover up their ignorance with statements that amount to something like this: "Social change is the result of all factors that enter into the production of social change," it is our belief that changes and discoveries come about through the operation of natural law. We have more to say about natural law in a subsequent chapter, but here we want to simply state that natural law operates to make possible important discoveries, like the discovery of the role of grandiosity, when they are most needed, and when the human race can make the best use of them.

Few will deny that the discovery of the direct cause of emotional and behavior problems is most necessary at this point in history when such problems are multiplying at an alarming rate. And there has been no time in history when so many need the kind of therapy that this discovery suggests. We believe that natural law operates with an awareness of these kinds of situations and operates to meet them, for, like many others, we believe that natural law is just another name for God or by what other name you desire to call the Intelligence or the Power that so undeniably and remarkably controls the universe.

Before going on to describe how we view the development of grandiosity in an individual's life, it is extremely important that the concept of grandiosity, as we use it in Natural Therapy, be fully and correctly understood. We are concerned about this, because it has been our not uncommon experience that some, who have read our first book, apparently have a difficult time precisely comprehending this concept.

Many apparently find it possible to understand it only in terms of an individual strutting around, showing off, calling attention to himself and his great accomplishments, and the like. We remember a professor at a school we attended, who walked out of the banquet hall, when he was introduced by a master of ceremonies who failed to prefix the professor's name with his "Doctor" title. Most people, even as the author and other students attending did, would call his behavior grandiose. Thirty years later we would not be so sure.

As some say of insanity and sanity, there is apparently only a fine line dividing at least the outward appearance of grandiosity and true self-esteem. And we have often advised students to answer anyone who calls them grandiose: "It takes one to know one!" So reread our description of grandiosity in an earlier section if you feel that you do not have that concept adequately trapped before going on.

THIS IS HOW WE VIEW THE ORIGIN
OF GRANDIOSITY

In fashioning Natural Therapy there were two questions that we had to answer: Why are some grandiose and others not? and, Why do some develop principally *emotional* problems, while others develop principally *behavior* problems?

Those that feel that the environment is the principal determinant of human behavior answer those two questions on the basis of the kind of conditioning the problem individuals received especially in childhood. However, studies of children born and reared in the same family, and of identical twins separated from birth and reared in different environments, do not allow for such easy explanation.

There is, however, a natural explanation, and it is the key to Natural Therapy for emotional and behavior problems. Hans Eysenck, Director of the Institute of Psychiatry at Maudsley Hospital in London, through rigorous scientific experimentation has produced a great deal of evidence (see his books listed in the references) to prove that all human beings are, personality-wise, somewhere on a continuum ranging from difficult-to-condition to easily-conditioned. He referred to the difficult-to-condition individuals as extraverts, and the easily-conditioned individuals as introverts; in between, of course, are the moderately-conditionable often called ambiverts. Apparently, variable conditionability determines the degree of extraversion-introversion.

Extraverts have been described as outgoing, sociable, impulsive, loud, carefree, aggressive, somewhat unreliable, happy-go-lucky, tough-minded, and optimistic. Introverts are said to be inwardly-directing, introspective, quiet, unassertive, reserved, careful, serious, controlled, very reliable, tender-minded, and pessimistic. Ambiverts apparently have approximately equal qualities of both, but in moderation. (We shall show later how the terms extravert and introvert themselves have led to a great misunderstanding of how an individual develops these kinds of personality traits.)

It is doubtful if there are any pure extraverts or introverts, and it is likely that everyone has qualities of both to some degree. The extravert overbalances on the extravert side, and the introvert on the introvert side. No one knows how many extraverts, introverts, and ambiverts there are in the American population, but our guess is that the distribution would follow somewhat a normal, bell-shaped curve, with approximately two-thirds of the population ambiverted, and the remaining third divided about equally between the extraverts and the introverts.

Eysenck also found that both extraverts and introverts are highly emotional. This high emotionality, of course, adds a high degree of interest and concern to whatever these individuals feel that they must do. We shall later describe the relationship between acquired grandiosity and this inborn high emotionality and its significance.

What we are primarily interested in here is the difference in conditionability found among people. How does an individual acquire his particular degree of conditionability? Eysenck describes it as hereditary and sees a possible relationship to the kind of reticular formation in the central nervous system with which an individual is born.

We find some good reasons why individuals should be born with different degrees of conditionability. If you are a believer in biological evolutionism, you would have to agree that variable conditionability in humans had to develop if the race was to progress or even to survive. If you believe in divine creationism, you would also have to agree that variable conditonability in humans would have to be included in the genes and chromosomes by the Creator if the race was to progress or even survive. Without individuals in every age who would have the courage to do daring things, as difficult-to-condition individuals can have, it is doubtful if humanity could progress or even survive for very long.

Without individuals in every age who would be concerned about the welfare of others, as easily-conditioned individuals can be, and who could also moderate the excessive daring of others, it is doubtful if humanity could progress or even survive for very long. And without large numbers of humans in every age who could support the endeavors of the other two kinds of people, and do so without excessive emotion or any great degree of compulsion, as moderately-conditionable individuals can, it is doubtful if humanity could progress or even survive for very long.

With such important roles to play in the progress and survival of humankind, it is also easy to understand why the easily-conditioned and the difficult-to-condition individuals were endowed by evolution or the Creator, whichever is your belief, with such a high degree of emotionality, insuring that they would go about their important work with a great deal of zeal and faithfulness. It is also easy to understand why the moderately-conditionable were endowed with only moderate emotionality, insuring that they could render the kind of steady and sometimes even monotonous and boring support that the work of the other two kinds of individuals needs to have if it is to succeed. It also explains, in addition, why it is often so difficult to motivate them to do the important work that they are by nature so well-equipped to do.

Now we are ready to determine why some individuals develop or acquire grandiosity and others do not, and why some of the grandiose develop principally *behavior* problems while other grandiose individuals develop principally *emotional* problems.

The easily-conditioned individual is highly impressed with only the ordinary care he is given as a child. He not only, like most people, thinks he is something special; he thinks he is extra-special. And, if his parents spoil and pamper him, as so many parents do these days in bringing up their children, he thinks he is super-special. Even if his parents neglect or abuse him, the little grandiosity he has already acquired because he has received at least enough care to enable him to survive, forces him to overcompensate, as Adler has pointed out, and his grandiosity soars nevertheless.

Unlike the easily-conditioned individual, the difficult-to-condition individual is only minimally influenced by what happens to him from without, so it makes little difference to him if his parents take care of him or neglect or abuse him. Only minimally influenced from without, he feels little restraint upon his felt needs and drives. And he begins to live primarily to have his needs and drives filled at any cost. This is another form of grandiosity. Thus, while easily-conditioned individuals and difficult-to-condition individuals react in opposite ways to conditioning from without, they both can end up as grandiose.

Incidentally, Camilla Anderson feels that everyone becomes grandiose by virtue of his very survival. And it is true that everyone acquires a degree of self-esteem, or at least self-interest, as a result of the fact that he received enough attention to insure his survival. However, this kind of self-esteem, which is characteristic of the moderately-conditionable individual, is just enough to insure that the individual will be interested in his own self-preservation, in caring for his basic needs. We prefer to use the term grandiosity only for those whose self-feelings are more grand.

It is now evident why the easily-conditioned individual develops significant problems primarily in the area of emotion, while the difficult-to-condition individual develops significant problems primarily in the area of behavior.

The easily-conditioned individual is highly impressed with the expectations others have of him and the demands made upon him from without. This factor, together with the grandiosity he has acquired, makes him feel that he has to be perfect and to perform perfectly. Of course, this also includes the idea that others must look up to him and cater to him, for, if they don't, this somehow mars the perfect life he feels he must enjoy. Such unrealistic and impossible expectations can never be fulfilled in this world, and whenever they fail to be fulfilled, he develops all sorts of emotional problems, ranging from anxiety and guilt-feelings to depression and even panic. The tension inherent in such emotional states produces a wide variety of physical symptoms which add to his misery.

The difficult-to-condition grandiose individual is mainly concerned with getting his drives and needs filled at almost any cost. His high emotionality compels him to push others aside and to ignore the rules to accomplish this. The result is that he has behavior problems, for his behavior is such that he has troubles with other people, with authorities, and with the law. He finds himself opposed, ostracized, and sometimes imprisoned. The inherent tensions also produce adverse physical effects.

It should also be mentioned that the ambivert or moderately-conditionable individual, who has characteristics of both the extravert and the introvert, but in more moderate form, does not develop grandiosity, as explained earlier. He develops a rather proper amount of self-esteem or self-concern, and thus feels only a moderate need to be perfect, to have his needs filled, and to have others cater to him. Of course, even this moderate need can be frustrated, and emotional and behavior problems do develop, but they also will be only moderate problems, and most such individuals are able to handle them. Others may feel the need for professional help, and it is with these that many professionals have some success, enough success apparently to keep them in business despite their consistent lack of success, as many recent studies indicate, with those whose problems are more difficult and more painful.

GRANDIOSITY PRODUCES HAVE-TOS

To understand this better it might be helpful if we consider certain aspects of what has become known in general as ego psychology. Many believe that Freud, who tried to explain all human behavior on the basis of the interplay between the so-called *id* (the basic instincts), the *ego* (what the individual thinks of as himself), and the *superego* (roughly equivalent to conscience), considered the *id* to be the most important of the three in determining behavior.

Beginning with Alfred Adler, however, who gave important consideration especially to individual life style, and
who on that account became known as the founder of *individual psychology,* and continuing through later psycho-
analysts, there has arisen a widespread interest in the ego,
or what the individual thinks of his self or himself as the
prime determiner of the form that individual behavior
takes or ought to take. Such a view is shared by existential
psychology, humanistic psychology, gestalt psychology,
and the like, which have come into prominence especially
in recent times.

Recently we were reminded of how prevalent ego psychology is even among the younger clergymen when we
met up with a former student of ours, who had recently
become interested in advancing his counseling knowledge
and skills. When we described our Natural Therapy to
him, the first thing he said was: "What does the client get
out of it for himself?"

To understand the rise and presence of have-tos or compulsion in grandiosity, one must have a real appreciation
of how a grandiose individual, consciously or unconsciously (though most often unconsciously), views himself or
herself. In grandiosity the self is the prime focus of attention in any situation. One writer described one of the
characters in his novel as a little country bounded on the
north, the south, the east, and the west by herself. That's
grandiosity.

To a grandiose person his own self is his most priceless
earthly possession, and his most important concern day in
and day out is to build a wall around it to protect it from
any possible harm. Almost every thought and action of a
grandiose person has something to do with the preservation of his ego.

From that point of view it should be easier to understand
that feelings of inferiority (which are really a prominent
symptom of grandiosity) are not really an evidence of a
weak ego. No one in his right mind would go around

defending and protecting that. If you insist that an individual with inferiority feelings is actually trying to protect his fragile ego, then we counter with the question: "If he is so concerned with protecting it, is that not an indication of his basic grandiosity?" There are a lot of people with feelings of inferiority that have accepted them and do not have any significant problems as far as they are concerned. You might say: "Oh, if he would really get rid of his inferiority feelings, he could be promoted in his job or be more outwardly successful, etc." But if he is not concerned about a lack of promotion or outward success, that is no problem for him. Only those who are *concerned* about their feelings of inferiority are grandiose, and they have developed have-tos thereby which cause their problems. In fact, it is the grandiosity and its inherent compulsions that have produced the concerns about feeling inferior in the first place.

To get an idea of what have-tos are really like and how they constantly drive and control the grandiose individual, consider, for example, a non-grandiose individual's interest in his physical welfare and safety. We have made the statement earlier that moderately-conditionable people, so-called ambiverts, have just enough self-interest to be concerned mainly about their physical self-preservation. We stated later that those who escape significant problems are those whose ego was developed just enough to make them interested in their physical self-preservation.

Consider for a moment, then, what these ordinary individuals do to preserve their physical life. They make certain that they eat and drink enough, get enough rest and sleep, work enough to earn money for food and clothing and shelter, brush their teeth fairly regularly (though you may find some that don't), wash their clothes, do the dishes, usually go to the doctor when they are ill, take their prescribed medicine, try to drive carefully, look both ways before crossing a street, keep away from open places and from under trees during lightning storms, and do a thousand other things day in and day out, year in and year out, all just to preserve their health and insure their continued physical existence. Even the weakest ego will induce an individual to stay on this treadmill of almost interminable activity toward that end.

Now consider what the grandiose person does, *in addition,* to preserve his or her physical existence. He or she is likely to do many or all of the following daily or frequently and most certainly with a great deal of gusto, precision, and slavish persistence: buy his food at a health food store, take vitamin supplements, keep up on the latest about proper diet, be overconcerned with his weight, indulge in monotonous daily jogging or other strenuous exercise, be concerned about the kind of house he lives in and the prestige of its location, make certain that the gas jets are turned off before leaving his house or going to bed, be careful about the kind of tooth paste he uses when he brushes his teeth several times a day if not also after every meal, avoid wearing the same underwear two days in a row, wash his hands many times during the day, rush to his doctor at the first sign of a strange or new pain, constantly scan traffic in all directions when driving and keep his right foot poised over the brake pedal, never miss taking his pills, watch every penny though at the same time spending dollars very foolishly, be greatly disturbed when overcharged, be certain to have "buyer's remorse" even when making a minor purchase, etc., etc.

In all this it is quite clear that a grandiose person is compelled or driven by his high ego to have a strong concern about anything that even remotely has or may have any possible relation to himself. Just as some wealthy person, even though he possesses enough funds to meet almost any possible material need that he may ever have, cannot enjoy the security that great wealth can bring, because he is always overconcerned that he could and might lose it, just so the grandiose person, who really possesses natural qualities that could produce the true self-esteem and concomitant self-confidence that such qualities can bring, is compelled by that grandiosity to be more concerned about just maintaining that grandiosity than with the enjoyment of all the more wonderful things that his special and natural qualities could bring.

In a recent college class in deviant behavior we were constantly trying to impress upon the members of the class that have-tos play an all-important part in the production of what some people regard as deviant behavior. On one of our field trips we took the class to a hospital whose alcoholism-rehabilitation unit had one of the highest reputations in our area. As we neared the end of a very fine presentation by the nurse in charge of the unit about the work being done there, we asked what was the most important factor in the personality profile of the alcoholic that was maintaining his alcoholism. And we watched with a great deal of satisfaction the smiles spreading over the faces of the students at her reply, the only reply, we felt, that could be made, if indeed that hospital was as successful with alcoholism as it was reputed to be; it consisted of only one word, but that is all it had to be: "Compulsion." She did not have to elaborate for this class, but she did add what the class already knew: "Alcoholics feel that they *have to* . . ." do this or that, have this or that, etc., etc. In our class that meant that alcoholics' real problem stems from the fact that they have developed a feeling of grandiosity about themselves. We say more about alcoholism in a later chapter, but here we use it to demonstrate again the have-to aspects of grandiosity.

The grandiose person is a driven person, forced unceasingly to be on the alert, to make use of every opportunity, to manipulate almost every person and every situation, to use every strategem, to pay almost any price — all in order to preserve his own high view and expectations of himself. When you hear people described as "living lives of quiet desperation," you can be certain that it is grandiose individuals that are being described, for a more apt description could hardly be found.

In fact, such people are sometimes compelled by their grandiosity even to deny reality, if necessary, to preserve their exaggerated egos. This is clearly seen among those whose grandiosity has reached such proportions that they call themselves Napoleon or Christ or some other prominent person. Once when attending a study session at a mental hospital we said to one of the inmates: "They tell us that you are the president of a bank." He quickly and excitedly replied: "The president of a bank? Why I own all the banks in the world!"

On another occasion, when we had gathered our weekly religion class together at the local state hospital near the church we pastored, we were telling some of the old Bible stories that they liked to hear. There was, however, one member of the group who always made certain to show us that he was superior to the rest of the group, usually appearing to be totally uninterested, and trying to impress us with his gross inattention by looking in every direction but ours. On this occasion he suddenly interrupted to proudly announce: "I was there when all that happened!" He just couldn't keep his grandiosity in check any longer.

The compulsions that are part and parcel of grandiosity are never so evident as when we see them binding individuals completely to themselves, so that they really can see no other but themselves. We are reminded here of the closing scene in Ibsen's play "Peer Gynt," when Peer Gynt observes that some inmates of a mental institution are "beside themselves". But the superintendent of the asylum replies:

> "Beside themselves? Oh no, you're wrong.
> It's here that men are most themselves —
> Themselves and nothing but themselves —
> Sailing with outspread sails of self.
> Each shuts himself in a cask of self,
> The cask stopped with a bung of self
> And seasoned in a well of self.
> None has a tear for others' woes
> Or cares what any other thinks."

What is it that compels an otherwise "good" person to

lie, to cheat, to rob, to embezzle, to bribe, to gossip, to deceive, to feel guilty, to feel inadequate, to be resentful, to be unfaithful, yes, even to murder? Only the have-tos that germinate and are fed and nourished by grandiosity. Not only the Davids and Sauls and Abrahams of Biblical days, but kings and princes and presidents and congressmen of our own day.

Without trying to be judgmental or to appear to be any more moral than others, we point you to what former president Nixon and many of his top associates, high in the realm of trusted public office in our nation, were willing to risk and to lose in order to maintain their own high estimate of themselves and of what they considered to be of such worth to themselves that they did what, in even their own now saner and more humble moments, they must find it hard to understand why they really did it.

While the focus of our first presentation of Natural Therapy was on grandiosity as the direct cause of significant emotional and behavior problems, and the present book has been designed especially to emphasize the have-to aspects of grandiosity, we could hardly escape jumping the gun a bit in the first part of the present book and mentioning our later discovery of the importance of the have-tos inherent in grandiosity. We have done this intentionally, because grandiosity's important influences in producing severe problems can hardly be fully understood without a full appreciation of the effects of the have-tos inherent in it. Of course, much more needs to be said about those have-tos, and we have reserved a great deal of space for that in later chapters.

We have thus far in this book set the stage for a fuller discussion of the role of have-tos by outlining in this chapter Natural Therapy's original view of the *cause* of significant problems in the development of grandiosity. We complete the setting of that stage in the ensuing chapter.

chapter **2**

*Natural Therapy
And The Solution to
Significant Problems*

KNOW YOURSELF!

Natural Therapy's first direction for the control of significant problems is the same as the age-old advice given already by the ancient Greeks; "Know thyself!" But the truth is that the very persons who need most to follow such advice are usually the very ones who do not.

It is the grandiose person, the one we described in the previous chapter, and the one who usually has the most significant problems, who fails to get to know himself well enough to get on top of problems. Not because such individuals are not aware of the importance of trying to ferret out all the elements that enter into the problem. Such individuals usually are preoccupied with doing that very thing.

Their difficulty, however, is that they are too grandiose to go to a counselor, for that would be a humiliating admission of some personal failure. They prefer to read books about their kind of problem, but the conflicting advice in such books usually doesn't help them much. In addition, being grandiose, they often believe that they really do know themselves, and they usually react favorably only to that kind of outside information that coincides with their own ideas about themselves.

To try to get to know one's self in such a situation — beset by one's own blinding grandiosity and perplexed by the conflicting theories of those on the outside who are supposed to know — is no simple task.

At this point it is important for the grandiose sufferer to discover only those characteristics about himself that will help him to understand why and how he developed his problems, and that also play an important part in their solution. In our insistence upon this narrow focus of this self-inventory, we are also pointing out that the eclecticism so characteristic of prevailing American therapy has no experimental evidence to support it and can only hamper this self-search.

Such eclecticism, which, broadly defined, holds that there are many different causes for problems and thus there can be many different solutions to them, only makes the task of knowing one's self almost impossible. While we can understand that prevailing American therapy's love affair with environmental determinism, which opens a Pandora's box of countless external influences that need to be considered, makes such a personal inventory almost impossible, we also point out that Natural Therapy's insistence on biological determinism, which, in the case of significant problems, can operate on the basis of "one cause and one cure" for such problems, narrows the self-search to inborn characteristics, and most importantly to degree of conditionability. Other natural characteristics do play a part, but, in our opinion, their particular roles are not important enough to be considered in this book, which already has many more important factors to deal with. One such characteristic, which some others believe is very important, is degree of intelligence. While agreeing that degree of intelligence does play a part in human problems, both in their origin as well as in their solution, we feel that its major role is that it increases or decreases the part that any other factors play in human problems. For example, and contrary to what one might expect, the higher the degree of intelligence, the more likely there will be problems and the more difficulty there will be in trying to overcome them. Actually, in the solution to your problem, which we shall describe in a subsequent section, the initial step will be to eliminate the many factors that appear to bear an important relationship to the problem, but which bear no significant relationship at all, except, unfortunately, only to prevent or at least delay the solution. While such factors may appear formidable and also of great number, we shall be able to eliminate them in one fell swoop as we, beginning already in this section, give them some momentum in that direction, by directing your attention to the very few characteristics that you have, that are really the ones that are responsible for the problem.

Take our word for it that this is where you need to start: discover the causes of your problem by first discovering yourself. We make that statement because you are probably like so many, who have significant problems, who want only to be saved from the results of their problem and are not really interested in their causes. There are many reasons for this, as we already pointed out in our first book. But problems are never really solved if we do not eliminate their causes, and full knowledge of those causes is the first step in that direction.

Do not protest that you have already made a diligent search for those causes, and perhaps even have paid a great deal of money to professionals who were supposed to be able to help you in that search, and you have come up empty. We have heard those kinds of protestations too often, and, in addition, we also for over thirty years were on that same kind of search ourselves, as we indicated earlier, for ourselves, for others, and also with others, with equally negative results. And it is our conclusion, which we can abundantly document, that such failure is due principally to the failure to begin, continue, and end that search almost entirely with a complete study of the individual who has the problem. As someone has wisely said: the self-conscious, paradoxically, need to be conscious of the self. We see already in the very next section how true all this is.

HOW CONDITIONABLE ARE YOU?

In Natural Therapy the type of conditionality in an individual is the key to understanding both the cause and the solution to human problems. It is the key, for one important reason, because it suggests an important reason why human problems, of the kind that concern you, are so difficult to solve. Prevailing psychotherapy, at least in America and Soviet Russia (you will soon be able to understand why there is such agreement in this matter between two widely differing nations), while recognizing variable conditionability among humans, does not find the type of conditionability of any great importance in the etiology of significant human problems.

We hold that this is the very reason why the representative approaches of these two nations have generally failed to solve such problems. They refuse, for the most part, to look for the origin of the problem in the individual, because it is their opinion that it is not the conditionability of the individual that causes the problem so much as it is that which does the conditioning.

Now see where that has led them. It has forced them to look at the sufferer as a more or less passive participant, and largely also a powerless one, in the most important aspects of his problem. Under those conditions they have already lost much of their ability to solve the problem. Very often the conditioning agent is no longer in existence, and even if it were, there is often little that can be done to eliminate or modify it. There are myriads of examples that could demonstrate this, but let us consider only, for example, the utter failure on the part of this approach to solve the crime problem by changing the conditioning environment (poverty, gangs, etc.) that, from their point of view, produces it. Not long ago, when we met with a representative of our state Attorney General, Evelle Younger, who had become interested in Natural Therapy, one of the first things we asked him was: "What has been the success of any programs to solve the crime problem in California based on environmental determinism?" The reply came without any hesitation: "Absolutely none."

Why would American psychotherapists be so determined to hold to their emphasis on environmental determinism, despite the great and increasing empirical evidence of the repeated failure of such an approach? Could it be that many of them would have to go out of business if it was generally held by their profession that significant problems had basically a genetic or biological cause, in which case, on the basis of the other ideas so many hold about human problems, they could only tell the sufferer, as in fact many of them are already doing, that they have to learn to put up with the suffering? Have you not noticed how increasingly many therapists are saying: "Anxiety is natural, so don't get so upset about it." This is partly true, but not usually for the kinds of problems that induce people to come to others for help. Most of such talk is, in our opinion, very often just a copout.

As far as Soviet psychology is concerned, the whole ideology behind Russian-type communism, which controls its psychology, is based on the idea that one can get one's needs satisfied by creating an environment that enables everyone in that same environment to have an equal opportunity to have his needs met through that same environment. If that sounds like an overemphasis on the environment, it really is, and that's exactly why communism, Russian-type at least, has not worked too well and never will. Despite the fact that the Soviets have had perhaps the greatest control over environment ever seen in the history of humankind, the resultant changes have been, updating Bulgakov, a prologue for only a few, and a select few at that, but an epilogue for very, very many, including some of their top talent.

We have gone a long way around to try to impress you with the fact that, no matter what you have been believing about yourself up till now, if you want to get on top of that important problem that is dogging you right now and up-setting your life, it is imperative that you have no doubt that it is your type of conditionability that is most inti-mately involved with it. And the best way that we can help you fully embrace that belief is to insist that the type of conditionability that is part and parcel of your being has not been acquired from, or even been significantly modi-fied by, anything outside of you. It's inborn, determined by your genes and chromosomes. And, for weal or woe, you are stuck with it.

Stuck with it? That's the way it may appear now. But, just to give you a little encouragement at this point, Natural Therapy is a way of changing inherited degree of conditionability from a rather painful liability into a most priceless asset.

We have found it advisable to give such encouragement at the very beginning of any attempt to implement the therapy, because we have usually found that the very dif-ferent approach of our therapy, as well as the fact that very often it appears to many to be very complicated and not too easy, tends to discourage some, especially those who have been battling their big problem for some time. Don't be discouraged! It all becomes more understandable, more clear, and, in fact, easier, as you follow faithfully each step that this book directs. If you ask: How long does it take to get in control of my problem?, the answer is: One step at a time. Keeping that always in mind, let's continue.

So the important question is: How conditionable are

you? That question cannot be fully answered until you also consider the conditioning agent, specifically whether it comes from within (from inner needs and drives) or from without (from the environment).

If you turn back to page 15 where we describe the characteristics of so-called extraverts and introverts, it might be simple for you to judge whether you are predominantly one or the other. If you can decide on this basis that you are an extravert, then you are difficult-to-condition by conditioning agents that come predominantly from without, but easily conditioned by inborn drives and needs from within.

If you decide on this basis that you are an introvert, then just the opposite is true — you are easily-conditioned from without, but difficult-to-condition from within. Now you are beginning to understand why the terms extravert and introvert are half right and half wrong, which may be one reason why prevailing American psychology, while admitting that there are indeed personality traits that might be described as extravert or introvert, points out that there appears to be a lack of consistency in such designations. Its apparent failure to seek or to discover why apparent inconsistencies do manifest themselves in the same individual has led them to throw the baby out with the bath water — to reject what to us is the key to a fundamental understanding of human behavior.

Of course, we believe that part of the evident inconsistency is due indeed to the failure to distinguish the differing sources of the conditioning agents, and why some are influenced more by one than the other. We have already tried to make this clear in the very first chapter, but we are trying to reinforce this truth also here, because it is important for you to fully understand this, if you are to understand your conditionability.

At this point, then, if you are able to classify your type of conditionability on the basis of what we have just been stating, then you are ready to go on to see just how this type of conditionability is determining your behavior. If you are still in doubt about what your type of condition-ability is, then you might have some skilled person admin-ister to you Eysenck's Personality Inventory, which, we feel, is a fairly accurate objective instrument for making such a determination.

Now, if either of the assessments described above, your own or the EPI, or both, appear to indicate that you pos-sess approximately equal amounts of both types of condi-tionability, don't let that upset you, for you have just join-ed the club, because, in our opinion, about two-thirds of the population is characterized by that kind of condi-tionability. The initial indication of such a finding is that either your problem is not as significant as you think it is, or it is due to some exceptional kind or degree of condi-tioning in some area of your life; perhaps the latter is responsible for the exaggeration in the former.

If indeed you do possess approximately equal amounts of both basic types of conditionability, then you are basi-cally an ambivert. We keep on using the term "basically," because it is likely that there are no individuals that are completely and purely either extraverted, introverted, or even ambiverted; individuals are most likely only *predom-inantly* of one of those three types. Perhaps one ought to imagine conditionability in individuals as a continuum or straight horizontal line, with extreme extraversion on one end and extreme introversion on the other, with ambiver-sion in the center. It might be helpful also to place a short vertical line in the exact center of the line, bisecting it, and indicating that this is the point of equal amounts of extra-version and introversion, so that whatever is on one side of that line is predominantly extraverted and whatever is on the other side is predominantly introverted. It must be remembered, of course, that the amounts of extraversion or introversion increase as one moves to the right or to the left of that center line. Thus even an ambiverted indi-vidual will most likely show some, if only minimal and almost insignificant amounts of, predominance in one direction or the other. Of course, it is also to be noted that, although such a continuum will indicate that there are different types of conditionability among humans, ranging from one extreme to its opposite, this is not to imply that this variability proceeds from one end to the other at equal rates. By this we mean to indicate again that it is not as though ten percent of the population is extremely extraverted, that is, from 91 to 100 percent that way, that the next ten percent are 81 to 90 percent extraverted, etc. It is our considered belief that, somewhat like a normal curve, extreme extraverts may compose about one-sixth of the population, extreme introverts about the same amount, while ambiverts would occupy the middle two-thirds of the area under the curve, or two-thirds of the population, some a little introverted, others a little extraverted.

Failure to recognize this variability in basic type of conditionability is the other reason, we believe, that American psychology has failed to recognize the importance of conditionability in human behavior. When submitting their data on all that they knew about individuals who were generally typed as extraverts and introverts to correlational or factor analysis, they claim to have found that these two variables are not independent, indicating therefore that each variable has some characteristic or characteristics that the other also possesses. For that reason, they have discarded these concepts as not important, or, at least, not viable in trying to solve human problems, for how is one really to know when, how, and to what extent each may be involved in the problem?

We would suspect that the real reason why these concepts have been generally ignored by American psychologists is again their preoccupation with environmental factors, for a thorough study of these concepts can lead only to the recognition of the independence of these two variables, just as we have described them in the previous paragraphs. Furthermore, if they had tested these variables in their relationships to influences from within and influences from without, they could have discovered almost consistent evidence of independence. Any lack of independence might appear where an intervening variable produced by exceptional and severe conditioning was also involved, although even in this case they are likely to fail to correctly assess the influence of such an intervening variable, again because of their almost-exclusive acquaintance only with the environmental factors in behavior.

If it appears as though we are taking many detours in trying to help you determine your type of conditionability, they are intentional ones. We have discovered that our constant brainwashing by environmental determinism, as well as our own grandiosity's compulsions toward wanting to believe it and thus find causes only outside ourselves for our problems, are formidable obstacles in the way of our acquiring the kinds of insights, into our real condition, that will lead us to adopt the kind of program to solve our problems advocated in this book. For intelligent and highly educated people they are no doubt the most formidable obstacles. In our psychology and sociology classes we, of course, place strong emphasis upon biological factors in human behavior, and we usually find a strong resistance against their acceptance. We have found that we had to produce more evidence than even the environmental determinists do to support their opposite theories. Those who have attended our classes in recent years will remember the so-called "goodies" of the day with which we usually began class sessions. These were generally designed to provide new evidence from current news items that supported our position. Thus, even when the subject matter for the day's class session left no opening for inserting biologically-derived evidence, we made certain through the daily "goodies" to continue to peck away at the rather solidly entrenched opposite views that had enjoyed about a twenty-year headstart among our class members. This explanation may help you understand the approach used in this book.

By this time the more astute among you have guessed that, even though we could say that, strictly for therapy, it is not altogether necessary that you agree that your conditionability is inborn, it is a great deal better for you if you do. In fact, we might as well admit that part of the reason for our deliberate silence about that was to try to delay any such idea on your part, to induce mainly those of you, whose grandiosity is so great that you have difficulty in giving any views opposite to your own a fair hearing, to read on at least to this point, where we have just about shot our wad in offering, within the little space available for it in this book, what we believe is sufficient insight, which may have at least allowed you to entertain the possibility or even probability of the genetic determination of your kind of conditionability.

The final weapon in our arsenal of evidence for biological determinism is, in our opinion, the most formidable one. It is one to which we are all quite vulnerable, especially when we are faced with making a decision in a matter that is of great importance but also, for us at least, does not seem to have the 100 percent conclusive evidence we usually like to have. It is similar to a situation recently described to us by an old friend, who is theologically astute, but who is trying to decide whether he ought to have his newborn child baptized, for he is not fully convinced of the Scriptural evidence for infant baptism. While he stated that he did not like the kind of motivation involved, he would be in favor of the child's baptism, "just to be on the safe side."

In a similar kind of approach, we now point out that, if you do opt for the biological view of conditionability that we are espousing, you will have a great deal more going for you, in your desire to whip your problem, than if you do not. This claim is not merely based on the fact that the opposite point of view has already had its day, in your attempts to conquer your problem through it, and has been found wanting. It is based primarily on all that is involved in a biological point of view that is utterly lacking in its opposite, not only to give you a more rational insight into your problem (yes, it is true), but also to mobilize *all* the forces of nature in your behalf. That's also another reason why we call it *Natural* Therapy.

The challenge that we really hold out to you, when we strongly urge that you look upon your conditionability as a biological heritage, is that, if you do so, we firmly believe that you will have gained a knowledge of the most important earthly reason why you are here on earth. Conversely, if you don't, you will have missed it entirely. And, lest you consider that kind of a statement merely excessive, though well-meaning, hyperbole, designed to make a final try at getting you to launch out on just one more psychological voyage into the deep, into areas previously uncharted as far as you are concerned, then slowly and with great deliberation follow the compass bearings we now supply.

If indeed your conditionability is already determined for you in your genes and chromosomes, there are two principal ways, generally accepted among humans today, by which this has come about — through biological evolution or through divine creation (some speak also of a theistic evolution, which in the final analysis turns out to be just one form of creationism). While we have a difficult time understanding how scientists, most of whom have to be, or at least ought to be, experts in statistical probability, can think in terms of any kind of "by-chance-only" evolution, or rule out completely the possibility or even probability of a divine creation variable and still remain scientifically objective, the concept of a biologically-determined type of conditionability is not only possible, but also quite meaningful, whether the biology involved is attributed to either evolution or a Creator.

If your type of conditionability is the product of evolution, then it must also be accepted that this product of natural selection or adaptation, by which evolution is said to operate, is a biological imperative by which humans are to be assisted in meeting their ongoing needs for progress and survival. If your type of conditionability is the product of the omniscience and omnipotence of a Creator, then it is equally designed for the same high purposes.

Now see what all this means to you! Your type of conditionability is designed to meet the most important earthly needs of humankind, to say the least. You see now at least one big reason, for opting for a biological origin of your type of conditionability, is that it is so important that it is involved with the progress and even survival of humankind. Would it not also be imperative that no outside human or even non-human factor should ever be able to condition such an important quality out of the individual or eventually out of humankind, or even be able to effect any appreciable modification of it? (Carried further, this idea may be extended to suggest that any tampering with genes and chromosomes, at least in these kinds of areas, might certainly be detrimental to human progress and survival.)

After all this you should be in a confident position now to determine your type of conditionability, and to do so with a great deal of anticipation. You may find that you are basically conditioned more by factors outside yourself and less by factors from within yourself, in which case you are classified by this book as basically an easily-conditioned individual (an introvert in Eysenck's or generally accepted terms). As such your problem is likely to be more emotional than behavioral, in the area of feeling more than of conduct, unless in rare instances the opposite is true, in which case some severe conditioning by some unusually strong drive or need from within is the likely cause. The fact that your problem is a significant one indicates generally that your conditionability in the direction indicated is a strong one. And do not be surprised that you are a highly emotional individual who feels this way, not so much because you have a big problem that you are very much concerned about, but mainly because of the type of conditionability you have.

Or, you find that you are basically conditioned more by factors that come from within yourself, from your drives and needs, and less by factors in your environment, in which case you are classified by this book as a basically difficult-to-condition individual (an extravert in Eysenck's or generally accepted terms). As such your problem is likely to be more behavioral than emotional, in the area of conduct more than of feeling, unless in rare instances the opposite is true, in which case some severe conditioning from the environment is the likely cause. The fact that your problem is significant indicates that your conditionability in the direction indicated is a strong one. You are also highly emotional, not essentially because of the severity of your problem, but principally because it is a necessary concomitant of your type of conditionability.

We wish we could supply a precise explanation of the physical operation that brings about the phenomenon of conditionability. Eysenck believes that it has some involvement with the reticular formation of the central nervous system. A number of investigators have also discovered some evidence of chemical action that may have important influences in those types of reflex in humans. Because of the difficulty of performing experiments related to such factors on living human beings, it may be some time before the precise explanations of how the body produces what is manifested as variable conditionability become available to us. While it is conceivable that someday, on the basis of such explanations, it may be possible to devise ways to modify or even change basic type of conditionability, it may not be wise to attempt to do so, except in extreme cases. At any rate, since that day may be a long way off or may never arrive, it is important for you to go on to complete the inventory of those characteristics that you have that enter importantly into your problem.

The knowledge of your type of conditionability and its

importance to you is basic. All other imformation about yourself that is important to know in connection with your problem stems from that, so the remainder of your task of self-discovery can be completed in short order.

HOW GRANDIOSE ARE YOU?

If you do not recall why your type of conditionability is one of the kinds that predispose you to develop grandiosity under certain environmental conditions, then turn back to the first chapter and refresh your memory. And as you look back into your own past, you will likely be able to see exactly how this all took place in your life.

This will reinforce for you the acceptance of the fact that you are grandiose, and that, under the circumstances, you could not have avoided it. So we shall spend no further time to convince you of the fact that you are grandiose at the present time, and that it is the direct or immediate cause of your problem, especially because your grandiosity produces in you the compulsions or have-tos that we described at length in the previous chapter.

There are principally two aspects of grandiosity that should be referred to at this juncture to further assist you in knowing yourself and how you relate to those areas that are involved in your problem. One of them has to do with the strength of your grandiosity. It has been our experience that one of the things that makes it more difficult for people to effectively use Natural Therapy is that they underestimate the strength of their grandiosity.

In this, of course, they have the have-to stemming from their very grandiosity to assist them. No one likes to admit that he or she is grandiose. It is also not uncommon for those trying to use Natural Therapy to become very skillful in seeing the grandiosity in others, even where they never saw it before. At the same time these very same people continue to overlook the devious ways in which their own grandiosity controls so many aspects of their own lives.

WHAT ARE YOUR NATURAL QUALITIES?

While we have already taken a great deal of time and space to help you discover the one natural quality, that you possess, that is all-important in Natural Therapy — your type of conditionability, when we speak of natural qualities here, we refer to all other qualities, that you have, that are directly related to it. What these special qualities are will depend upon whether you are basically easily-conditioned (an introvert) or difficult-to-condition (an extravert). We have listed the special characteristics that each of these two types of individuals have on page 15, and you need only to refer to that page and to review for yourself those particular qualities that are listed under your type.

It is also to be noted that, besides these qualities, you also have other natural qualities that are not directly related to your type of conditionability, qualities like high intelligence, physical strength or endurance, artistic skills, and countless others, many of which you may not even be aware of. For this reason, it would be a good idea to maximize your knowledge in this area by taking one of the several very good aptitude tests available through many counseling agencies, public or private. The more of these kinds of additional natural skills that you can discover in yourself, the better for you.

Finally, while a knowledge of all your natural skills is very important, a knowledge of your acquired or learned skills can also be important. Such acquired skills are learned only because you also possess the natural qualities that make it possible. However, this does not make them less important; in fact, in some cases, they may be more important.

Furthermore, once you know what your natural qualities are, you should also consider how they might be used to enable you to develop other skills and qualities, which might be looked upon as extensions of natural qualities.

As you might suspect, there is more involved in all this than just becoming acquainted with all the qualities and potential qualities that you may have. Implicit in this search is the idea again that, because you have those qualities through inheritance and not through conditioning by the environment, they must have special importance. And unlike qualities that are acquired solely through conditioning from the outside, the old reminder to "use them or lose them" does not apply to them, for you really can never lose them. This, then, suggests that whatever agency produced them (whether in your belief it was evolution or a Creator), you have them primarily for purposes that have to do with the progress and survival of humankind.

We're sure that by now you are beginning to realize what Natural Therapy is really all about. While we hear a lot being said these days about nature, there is little doubt that so many do not really understand all that the term "nature" implies, especially for them. Most people think immediately about the world of nature all about them in the form of the grass and trees and animals and streams and the like. And somehow they do not usually conceive of themselves as any real part of all that. Most importantly and unfortunately, they do not seem to realize that the same laws that apply to nature apply equally to them.

So the human problem really comes down to two important failures: the failure to know who we are and the failure to be what we are. Thus far, we've tried to help you understand who you are. What follows is designed to overcome the second failure.

BE YOURSELF!

We are well aware of the fact that much of prevailing American therapy gives the same advice, but most people find it quite difficult to carry out in the ways that are implied by prevailing therapy. One of the difficulties is trying to decide which self, or which part of one's self, one ought to try to be, for there is also quite general agreement that humans consist of many selves, or, to put it more simply, hardly anyone is a totally integrated person, meaning that almost no one has every aspect of himself operating in perfect harmony. The question then is: What aspect of the self ought to predominate and also keep all the other aspects in line?

This is the problem, as we see it, with a very popular movement in today's psychology which emphasizes the importance of being a *self-actualized* person. If this adjective refers to the importance of developing one's potential to the maximum possible (an ideal with which few would disagree), there is still this important and over-ruling consideration to be dealt with: Which self is to be actualized? If each aspect of the self is to be maximally ac-tualized, one aspect is sure to find itself warring with its opposite. One would probably have to settle for one aspect of the self becoming predominant and whipping the other aspects into line, thus achieving integration at some level or other.

The problem in the latter case would resolve about deciding which aspect is to be given priority. And here, since value-systems differ from person to person, there would follow the inevitable clash with another trying to self-actualize in the same way but coming from a different value-system.

When Natural Therapy advises people with significant problems to be themselves, it means something quite definite and unmistakable. That advice is built upon the knowledge previously acquired about who one is in terms of one's natural qualities, especially one's degree of condi-tionability by external influences. To be one's self, in Natural Therapy's terms, is simply to try to use one's natural qualities primarily for the purposes that nature in-tended — the survival and progress of humankind.

Immediately you see how Natural Therapy's way of be-ing one's self differs from so much of prevailing therapy's ways, which usually emphasize the importance of being one's self *for* one's self, for one's own advancement, self-interest, and self-aggrandizement, and exclusively so. We are not saying that Natural Therapy is suggesting that we be ourselves not at all for ourselves. Actually, as we shall see later in this book, those who practice Natural Therapy are the greatest beneficiaries of its great results, and at no time does it expect us to act unselfishly.

Prevailing American therapy seems to foster the idea that everyone else is better off if each individual does his own thing for himself, implying thereby that in that way everyone is meeting his own needs, leaving no other needs to be satisfied. The important error in this kind of thinking is that no one is able to get his own needs at all adequately satisfied by trying to do so only through actualizing himself for himself.

Now, it would be great if you could at once put all your natural qualities, as well as all the additional abilities you acquired through them, into immediate operation as completely and effectively as you will certainly be able to do eventually to solve your problems. But at this point you must be made aware of the obstacles that for now prevent you from doing so, and learn how to remove them once and for all. You can truly be yourself by following the three directions in the following sections.

It is extremely important to know that there is one great obstacle that impedes the whole program, and which can only be adequately controlled in the later stages of the program — your thinking habits, which form the acting habits that are the ultimate target of Natural Therapy. At this point we can only strongly encourage you to keep aware of them, and to do your very best to keep them in line, until you can finally gain a firmer and more permanent control over them.

Because you are aware of that part of your problem and have learned a temporary way of dealing with it, you can now begin to pick off the less important, though still formidable obstacles, that need to be removed, one by one, if you are finally to reach your final goal — the removal of your problem and the prevention of any future significant problems in your life.

FIRST, SWITCH THE FOCUS TO THE REAL PROBLEM!

Earlier we stated that many years ago we realized that people with problems apparently could not get themselves off their hands, that they walked in a hall of mirrors, seeing themselves no matter in what directions they looked. We did not know why this apparently universal phenomenon among people with problems occurred, nor did we know how to eliminate it and thus solve the problem.

Of course, like most therapists, we were successful for a time in helping individuals sidetrack it and escape it temporarily. We sent them to doctors, and they received pills. We sent them off on vacations. We created jobs for them in the church's program. We told them to volunteer for charity work, to collect stamps, to have a little fun, to get a divorce, to mix with people, etc. While we have no idea how many permanently solved their problems by following that kind of advice, we suspect that none of them really did. Of course, we also tried to dig into their past to determine what early experience might be responsible for their undue preoccupation with themselves, but, because we did not really know what we were looking for, that search invariably also proved fruitless.

We cite these experiences to illustrate that solutions to problems are doomed to failure from the very beginning when they are not applied to the real cause of the problem. When people with problems see only themselves, no matter in what direction they look, that in itself is not all bad. In fact, it is good in one special sense. The real problem is that, when they see themselves, they see only their pain, their guilt, their frustration, their hostility, their headache, their disappointment. All this covers up the unseen problem that is producing the highly visible symptoms of the problem upon with their eyes are riveted.

The individual suffering from an emotional problem, for example, may be concerned only with his guilt-feeling and the tensions that accompany it. The individual with a behavior problem may be concerned only with his inability to get along with others and the frustrations and tensions inherent in such a situation. Under such circumstances a vicious circle is usually set up. Emotional problems produce tensions which create additional emotional problems. Behavior problems produce reactions that create additional behavior problems. To break this circle it is necessary to stop the ceaseless preoccupation with the emotional and behavior problems and their physical effects, and to concentrate on the real problem, the problem that produced them — grandiosity.

In our previous book we described at length how to go about switching the focus to the real problem. Basically we advised there that, when an emotional or behavioral problem and its accompanying physical symptoms arise, the individual experiencing them should not try to fight them but accept them for what they really are — not really as frightening or disturbing as they seem to be, but mere manifestations of the grandiosity the individual has acquired.

Thus when an emotional or behavior problem and its physical effects engulf you, you should immediately remind yourself that they are only reactions produced by an acquired grandiosity. In this way you shift your attention away from something with which you found yourself unable to cope to something which is not terrifying, and which you can learn to control. This shift of focus should be attempted at the very first inkling that an emotional upset is coming on, or at the very first awareness of an arising temptation to act improperly.

If something like this is not done, here are examples of what usually happens. An individual who feels a pain in his stomach, which has been produced by the tensions associated with his emotional problems, becomes fearful about the pain, creating additional emotional problems and preventing him from dealing with his real problem — grandiosity. Similarly, an individual who feels hostility to others who oppose his unacceptable behavior strikes out blindly at them, thus producing additional behavior problems and preventing him from dealing with his real problem — grandiosity.

In reminding yourself that your real problem is grandiosity, you can also be assisted by realizing that this grandiosity has been produced basically by the kind of conditionability with which you were born. This should eliminate any self-blame that may arise when grandiosity is discovered.

In addition, this should also eliminate the blaming of others. Of course, as we shall show in a later chapter, such grandiosity could have been prevented by parents, but the fact is that parents generally have been ignorant of the part that conditionability plays in personality development.

Thus self-blame and blaming of others should be eliminated from your thinking, for, in truth, no one is to blame. Eliminating any blame eliminates both guilt-feelings and resentment and facilitates the taking of the important first step in Natural Therapy — the acquiring and maintaining of a focus on the real problem.

When you remind yourself that your real problem is your grandiosity, then you can, at least temporarily, control the escalation of your problem or eliminate it momentarily. But, until grandiosity is properly dealt with, thoughts will continue to arise within you, again and again initiating an emotional or behavioral problem and its accompanying physical symptoms. For that reason, Natural Therapy suggests the following second important step.

SECOND, CHALLENGE EVERY MANIFESTATION OF GRANDIOSITY!

In our previous book on Natural Therapy we suggested

what is technically described as a cognitive behavior modification program to counteract any manifestation of grandiosity. Some of the ideas used there have been suggested by Albert Ellis' Rational-Emotive Therapy, which has been used with a great deal of success. For example, in Ellis' therapy, when someone is emotionally upset, it is because he feels that what has happened or will happen is awful, terrible, and catastrophic; to overcome his emotional problem he is to tell himself instead that nothing is really that bad, and that he is only exaggerating the importance of what has happened or will happen.

While Ellis does not specifically say so, to our knowledge, what he is doing in his therapy is that he is trying to reduce the grandiosity of the individual, which is producing his exaggerated view of his problem. In Natural Therapy we increase the value of Ellis' approach by helping the sufferer to see that he feels as he does only because of his grandiosity, thus eliminating some of the mystery and terror from the situation (with a corresponding reduction in the exaggeration of the problem), and paving the way for the elimination of this and any future problem by working on the modification of grandiosity.

After taking the first step in Natural Therapy, which consists, in effect, of recognizing, amid all the other symptoms also experienced, that grandiosity is the real problem, you extricate yourself from the vicious circle that perpetuates your problem. When emotional and behavior problems and their physical symptoms arise, you have learned to say to yourself: "It's only my grandiosity."

But, because it *is* grandiosity, it now needs to be controlled, for, unless it is, the problems and their tensions assert themselves again and again, to the point where you may find that reminding yourself that it is only grandiosity doing its dirty work becomes less effective and consequently is resorted to less and less.

This second step in Natural Therapy is designed to help you to begin to control grandiosity. It does so by asking you to learn to gain control over your thoughts. In thinking you are merely talking to yourself, and, unless you counteract what you say to yourself, you convert what you say into some kind of action.

Now the grandiose person is one who has developed the habit of repeating some things to himself that are just not entirely in line with reality. We don't mean that he is irrational. We mean that his grandiosity distorts reality just enough to cause him problems. In general, the easily-conditioned grandiose person tends to exaggerate the importance of what happens to him, while the difficult-to-condition grandiose person tends to minimize the importance of what happens to him. It's a little more complicated than that, but let that suffice to serve our present purposes.

Thus, if you are experiencing an emotional problem or feel one coming on, then, after putting a temporary stop to it by telling yourself that it is only your grandiosity acting up, use that brief interlude to listen in to yourself to determine what you are saying to yourself. Then quickly tell yourself that you are exaggerating the matter, that the situation is not as bad (sometimes also not as good) as you have been telling yourself it is. Challenge your thoughts (self-talk) in that way.

Similarly, if you are experiencing a behavior problem or are tempted to behave in an unacceptable manner, then, after putting a temporary stop to it by telling yourself that it is only your grandiosity leading you by the nose, use that brief interlude to listen in to yourself to determine what you are saying to yourself. Then quickly tell yourself that you are minimizing the harm you are doing, that the whole matter is more serious than you have been telling yourself it is.

Such challenges, consistently made, will serve to keep your problems under some control. But grandiosity is still around, and will resurrect old problems and create new ones. So, sooner or later it needs to be eliminated or at least significantly modified. The next procedure has been designed to do just that, and it is the heart of Natural Therapy.

THIRD, MASTER GRANDIOSITY BY MASTERING YOUR HAVE-TOS!

We have just suggested how to challenge the wrong kind of thinking (self-talk), the kind that produces problems. Now we suggest ways to form that habit of thinking (speaking to one's self) correctly and to prevent thereby the development of problems.

Up till now you have been using many of your characteristics principally for your own self-interest and self-aggrandizement, unknowingly insuring the continuation of your grandiosity and their accompanying destructive have-tos. Now, again using several cognitive behavior modification techniques, Natural Therapy advises you to remind yourself daily, and as often as possible, that you need now to use those same characteristics primarily to serve others and to improve the lot of humankind. In other words, change your destructive have-tos to beneficial want-tos.

If you are one who has principally emotional problems, then you are likely to be one who is overserious, concerned, reliable, careful, pessimistic, reserved, quiet, unassertive, controlled, tender-minded, introspective, etc. You have been using these characteristics almost exclusively to maintain your own grandiosity. You are overserious about any threat to yourself; you are concerned almost entirely about your own welfare; you use your reliability to make certain that you will always succeed and thus induce others to think highly of you; you are careful to avoid anything that will detract from your feelings of superiority; you use your pessimism to insure that you have considered all the dangers in a situation which might harm you; you are reserved to make sure that others will not get too close to you in order to avoid the contempt that familiarity often brings; you are quiet and unassertive so as not to do or say anything that might detract from the high opinion you feel others must have of you; you are tenderminded, not so much because you truly sympathize with others, but mostly because you are conscious of how terrible it would be if a similar evil happened to you; you are introspective to make certain that your conduct is always perfect, mostly in the eyes of others.

Now you want to learn to get yourself off your hands and master your grandiosity and its have-tos by reminding yourself daily and often to use these characteristics primarily in the service of others. Tell yourself over and over again that you must now use your overseriousness and concern primarily to be interested in helping to fulfill the needs of others; to use your reliability primarily to insure that the needs of others are met; to use your carefulness primarily to do the best job you can do in helping others; to use your pessimism primarily to make sure that nothing should go wrong in your efforts to help others; to use your tendermindedness primarily to have such sympathy for the needs of others that you will be led to help those in any need; to use your tendency toward introspection primarily to insure that you are doing what you can do to serve others.

If you are one who has problems that are principally behavioral then you are one who usually is outgoing, sociable, impulsive, loud, carefree, aggressive, unreliable, happy-go-lucky, toughminded, and optimistic. You, too, have been using these characteristics almost exclusively to maintain your own grandiosity. Remember your grandiosity consists of your feeling that you must (have-to) get your drives and needs fulfilled at any cost, so you use your outgoingness and sociability to get others to help fill your needs; you use your impulsiveness to prevent the rise of any thought of adverse consequences, which might deter you from your need-filling ventures; you use your loudness to get your need for attention from others filled; you use your carefreeness to brush aside anything that might prevent you from doing what you want to do to fill your needs; you use your aggressiveness to go after whatever you feel you need to have and do so with a great deal of drive; you use your unreliability to prevent others from becoming dependent upon you; you use your happy-go-lucky attitude to fill your need to feel that everything is always going all right for you; you use your tough-mindness to walk over others to get what you want; you use your optimism to maintain your confidence that all will work out all right no matter what you must do to get your needs filled.

Now you want to remind yourself daily and often to use these same characteristics primarily to serve others. Tell yourself to use your outgoingness and sociability primarily to determine what the needs of others are; your impulsiveness primarily to act quickly when the need to help others arises; your loudness primarily to call attention to the needs of others; your carefreeness primarily to take chances in order to help others; your happy-go-lucky attitude primarily to take in stride any failures in your attempts to help others; your tough-mindedness primarily to override any opposition to your attempts to help others; your optimism primarily to undertake difficult ventures to help others.

In general, whatever the type of your conditionability, whether your problem is primarily emotional or behavioral, you want now to remind yourself daily, and often during each day, to convert the use of any of your qualities or characteristics from primarily maintaining your grandiosity to primarily promote the welfare of humankind. And not only remind yourself so often to do so, but *to also embark upon a program of actively doing so.* In our previous book we suggested the use of behavior modification methods also to assist in putting such a program into actual daily practice gradually and regularly. You might profitably follow also that suggestion.

This entire procedure of now working primarily in the

interest of others, while it is the most important aspect of Natural Therapy, is also the most difficult. It can be initiated most easily by showing the proper interest in the welfare of those in the immediate family. It also has the additional advantage in that, when you fail now and then to do what you need to do, family members will generally overlook it, and thus lessen the trauma of such failure. On the other hand, family members may be too sympathetic and thus lower the kind of expectation of improved conduct on your part too much. So, by no means should it stop there. In addition, helping family members is often like helping yourself, for your family members are usually an extension of yourself. It is essential that any program of helping others should extend from the home as far as possible — even to strangers. And always remember, it must always be primary.

There is little danger that such activity will be overdone to the point of ignoring your own welfare. Remaining grandiosity or the newly-acquired proper amount of self-esteem will usually serve to avoid that. It is also true that you cannot help others unless you have also taken proper care of your own needs. To help others as much as you can also requires that you maximize your own natural potential, developing your natural qualities as much as possible. In this way and for this purpose, we are in some agreement with those who believe in self-actualization. At the same time, some interest in others is necessary.

Of course, doing things primarily for others does not mean that you must always permit others to walk all over you, or push you around. Though you may need to permit that to happen to you now and then, or maybe even often, there are other times when you can help others best when you actually get tough with them, and actually oppose what they are doing.

And we certainly do not mean that you should help others for the purpose of manipulating them for your own interests, something that grandiose persons do constantly, often without even realizing it. Nor do we mean mere "do-goodism" — a *token* interest in the welfare of others. We mean a genuine service that promotes the general welfare of humankind, and the welfare of specific individuals. Opportunities for such service abound everywhere.

When you render such help and service, your grandiosity is bound to decrease. In fact, something unusual happens: your false pride is replaced, not with the absence of any pride (no one could survive that), but with a true pride, the kind that results from worthwhile accomplishment.

No longer will you despise yourself; you have acquired a true self-regard (we made sure that we did not state self-love — you will understand why later). You who are suffering from emotional problems will acquire something you vainly sought before — the genuine esteem of others. You who are suffering from behavior problems will acquire something that you vainly sought before — the cooperation of others for the best kind of fulfillment of a greater number of your legitimate drives and needs. Both of you will function as nature intended. Both of you, in fact, will become what you erroneously thought you were before — truly superior persons.

While this concludes our brief summary of our first book, embellished considerably with the kinds of background information that we omitted from it, and slightly updated with the inclusion of some preliminary information about the have-to phenomenon, we do not advise that anyone try to use the therapy until after reading and digesting this entire present book. We know, from the responses to our first book, that a great many get turned on by the therapy from even less knowledge about it than we include in this and the previous chapter. And, we may add, many have received a great deal of help just from that.

Perhaps such eager response is due to the sheer novelty of its approach. Most other therapies today, except for the very far-out ones, usually proceed from common approaches that have existed for a long time. Transactional Analysis, for example, is neo-Freudian, and, if that were generally known, it would not have received such an initial response. But now people are finding that it is only as effective as neo-Freudianism, and it is understandably losing popularity.

So also Natural Therapy appears to be a brand new approach, that seems to be coming from an altogether new direction. While certainly, when compared with prevailing therapies of the past fifty years, it appears to be 100% different, and it is. Yet, as we indicate in chapter four, the oldest religions have been advocating something similar for several thousand years. That's why we have called it "an old yet new therapy." It's as old as natural law, which even predates humanity.

Unlike other therapies, however, Natural Therapy, as we stated at the very outset of this book, has always been around, which says something about its reliability and validity. And a great many people evidently sense that. It has the ring of truth, and we find people eager to plunge into it, even as some of you may find yourself right now.

But you want to go about this with all the knowledge about it that you can acquire. That will make it all easier for you and bring better results. We think that what we add in the rest of this book can bring a great deal of additional knowledge that will achieve such results. So, don't stop now. Read on with high expectations of what's still ahead for your more effective implementation of the therapy for your own special problems.

chapter **3**

Feedback
And Further Research

NATURAL THERAPY RECEIVES
INITIAL ASSESSMENT

Though the first book was not highly publicized or promoted for various reasons, mostly because of our own great ignorance about book publishing and promotion, but probably also because of a rather unconscious fear on our part that our therapy was too different and too tough to receive any great acceptance either from professionals in counseling, or from those who really needed the therapy, we had the gut-feeling that we really had something whose time had arrived. And, sure enough, it wasn't long before a number of people sought us out to give us their reaction.

Some of them just read the book and wanted to talk about it. Others both read the book and attempted to use the therapy for their problems and wanted to tell us about it. In addition, we sent copies of the book to prominent behavioral scientists, who were among the few whose work was really helping people with significant problems. The reactions and comments were all quite favorable, and, in some cases, even ecstatic. All this gave us enough courage to "come out of the closet" and to openly confront people with it in every possible way.

SEMINARS GAVE US EARLY FEEDBACK

Anyone who has ever been a relative unknown in any field of endeavor can understand how difficult it usually is to get any kind of adequate hearing for any new approach, and this is especially true in the field of therapy, which, over the years, and especially in recent ones, has witnessed the promotion of such an amazing number and variety of novel approaches, many of which have little to recommend them, that one usually has either to be well-known (no matter for what reason), to water down one's therapy to make it easy enough that many people will give it a try, or at least to publicize it in appropriate ways.

We made a kind of compromise by beginning our open promotion of Natural Therapy through seminars that were directed toward fellow Lutherans in West Coast cities from San Diego to Seattle. We made no attempt to highly publicize them for several reasons, the most important of which was to avoid anything that might cheapen the therapy in the eyes of anyone, or compromise its basic integrity and legitimacy. Thus, we were also practicing the therapy in the ways we sought to confront as many people with it as we could. In the long run, as Natural Therapy itself both proclaims as well as demonstrates, its interests would be served best by strict adherence to that principle.

While we hesitated to charge for attendance at these early seminars, some of our knowledgeable friends persuaded us that offering them for free would indicate to many that the therapy wasn't really worth much, though these same friends also shook their heads when we told them that the price we decided to charge would include a free copy of the book, which normally sold for 75% of the price of admission. But, in retrospect, this again demonstrated the validity of the Natural Therapy way, for apparently this admission price, though small, held the attendance down to a size where almost everyone attending had an opportunity to ask questions, and, perhaps even more important, it probably attracted those who were suffering enough, or interested enough to pay a price to find out more about it, and these were the kinds of people we were especially interested in attracting.

And we received some important feedback in the process. Some of it helped to assure us that the spiritual basis for the therapy was apparently unassailable, for we were able to give adequate replies to some in these audiences of primarily Lutheran people who had questions about it, including some pastors and professors. In the chapter that follows we include a consideration of some religious concerns.

In general, the seminars, coming as they did only about a year after the first book made its appearance, gave us the kinds of assurances, that we needed especially at that time, that the therapy could hold its own when exposed to scrutiny by those who are especially interested in such things, and no doubt also by those who are also highly knowledgeable in this area, for the seminars were also attended by some who were professional psychologists and counselors.

Aside from these kinds of feedback favorable to the therapy, we did also discover that, because those attending them had not read the book beforehand or ever really used that kind of therapy, we received from them no indication of how well the therapy worked. This was a little surprising to us, for we were convinced that the basic principles of the therapy were in high agreement with the kind of religion that Lutherans professed to believe. One by-product of this kind of feedback from the seminars, however, was our important decision to research this phenomenon, which has eventuated in the important discoveries revealed in the next chapter, which religious people should find especially relevant to their significant problems.

FEEDBACK CAME FROM COUNSELING

In addition to the seminars described above, we also accepted invitations to speak to various interested groups.

Some who attended wanted us to give them private counseling. In addition, we were receiving requests from those who lived at a distance, but who had read our book and wanted us to counsel them personally, even if only by mail or phone. While we were quite occupied with so many other activities, we agreed to accept a few of those requests, the ones that were related to some very difficult problems, even though the ones that were to be carried on by phone or mail were accepted only after we outlined the handicaps of working under such an arrangement. In addition, we insisted that we would take no remuneration, for we felt that in counseling on the basis of this different approach we were receiving as much as we were giving.

In these private counseling experiences we received feedback that was much more specific than the kind we received from speaking to groups. Perhaps the most consistent was the observation that the therapy was "so hard," or even "too hard." We should have expected those kinds of reactions, for, in our description of the grandiosity behind significant problems, we certainly had made it quite clear that grandiose people feel that things should be easy for them. These early reactions helped to confirm for us the idea that grandiosity certainly was the direct cause of such problems, but now we were beginning to realize also how powerfully it can control people.

In addition, it also became clear to us that grandiosity leads some people to believe that they know better, for some we were counseling evidently felt that they could skip some of the important steps they needed to take to receive help. Either we had not sufficiently impressed them with the importance of particular steps, or, more likely, they felt they could take some short cuts (because they were more intelligent ?). As a result we felt we had to impress them more with the importance of following each step outlined in the therapy. It got to the point where we had to tell some of them quite firmly that, when they were apparently not getting the kinds of results from their use of the therapy that they thought they should be having, they should promptly sit down again and carefully read over the book. Invariably they found that this was all that they had to do to get the kinds of results the therapy promised.

If we had to select two of the most important directions that many were failing to use, or to use properly, it would have to be the direction about how to put a quick stop to any feeling that an emotional upset or temptation to behave improperly was coming on, and the ultimate direction to use natural qualities primarily for the welfare of others. It's interesting that these two should be the most important ones in many ways, the first being a specific way to stop the problem from getting early control, and the other the final way to prevent it from even starting up again at all. The first is a temporary stop gap, and therefore most important especially in the early stages of using the therapy for the problem. The last is the ongoing activity that is an effective therapy for the problem, and becomes even a way of life that prevents future problems from developing.

FEEDBACK FROM STUDENTS

Our teaching of sociology, psychology, and anthropology at several state and private universities and colleges, both on a full-time as well as part-time basis, was very important in the development of Natural Therapy, and we continued part-time teaching, wherever possible, even after our first book appeared. Not only did this give us an opportunity to acquaint the students with this new development in the subjects that we taught, but it also enabled us to test out some of its principles among those who had both an academic as well as a vocational and possible future professional interest in it.

In our teaching we had always known about the importance of knowing as much as possible about those whom we tried to teach. Those who attended our classes in Educational Psychology would testify that we tried our best to get across the idea that the two most important psychological principles of successful teaching are: Know yourself, and know your students! Know them, of course, principally as to their natural qualities and how they are using them (the latter being evident by the presence or absence of grandiosity).

So it has been our custom in recent years to administer, at the beginning of each course, objective tests that seek to measure these two components in the class members, mostly for our own use in being a better teacher in that course. Such testing has also yielded some very helpful information also for updating of Natural Therapy, and we are grateful to the students that took those tests even though they were optional for the course.

These testings furnished corroborating evidence for some of the key ideas included in Natural Therapy. We had claimed that religious people were almost invariably of the easily-conditioned (introverted) type, and these testings remarkably demonstrated this. In addition, we had also claimed that some individuals of one basic type of conditionability sometimes displayed significant problems that were more characteristic of the opposite type, but that this was the result of some very severe conditioning in the particular area in which the uncharacteristic problem occurred. We felt that the failure to understand this phenomenon was one of the important reasons why American psychology in general has overlooked the importance of basic conditionability in problem-behavior.

While we administered these tests for other reasons, and we also had announced that we were not inviting our students to come to us for counsel just because we were administering tests that related in some ways to problems, some did approach us for counsel for specific problems, and in the process we did discover a few of those uncharacteristic problems. On the basis of our theory about this phenomenon, we probed the area of the problem, and each time we discovered some severe and prolonged conditioning in the past that could adequately account for it. It was also discovered in such counseling that, if the individual had other significant problems, they were always in the direction expected with their degree of conditionability.

These affirmations of important Natural Therapy theory, besides bringing a great deal of relief to some students who were greatly perplexed by apparent important inconsistencies in their life, also led us to bring our students more and more into the further development of the therapy. We exposed them to Natural Therapy's principles whenever the theories in our courses related to them, and they become a fine sounding-board, for certainly they could evaluate them from a more unbiased view than we could.

We even involved them, in a course in Deviant Behavior and Control, in the highly relevant development of a Have-To Inventory, which we will describe in greater detail later. With the input of so many who were not as unobjective about all this as their instructor was, we were not surprised that, when our completed Inventory was subjected to a Kuder-Richardson Reliability Test, it came up with a highly respectable score of .917.

FEEDBACK FROM READERS

We've already mentioned the fine feedback from those who read our first book and whom we took on for counseling. There were many other readers who contacted us for other reasons, all of whom helped to confirm through their own experiences what we had written about. It was not uncommon for people to seek us out, phone us, and say something like this: "You don't know me, but I read your book, and you described me so perfectly." They would often go on to describe how much they were suffering, and, even though we did not hear from some of them again, we like to think that they must have been helped by putting the therapy into practice. No one has ever told us that the new therapy did not work, while many have said that it did. When only a few have told us that *apparently* the therapy does not work for them, we have always found that either they did not fully understand it, or they were not practicing it properly.

It was good to learn that many thought that we knew what we were talking about when we tried to describe the kinds of problems for which Natural Therapy was designed. That alone would give people an additional incentive to give the therapy a try. But, in addition, there was another bonus for us in this type of feedback. After we had put Natural Therapy together for the first time and published it, we took occasion to speak to others about it whenever possible, and now we realize that, for some, our button-holing them and monopolizing the conversation with it must have been very boring. Sometimes we became a little disappointed at their apparent lack of interest or response, but now we realize that such individuals just don't have the kinds of significant problems that make them interested in what we're trying to get across to them. That's something good to know.

Actually this has great importance in our interpersonal relationships, about which we will say much more later. To give just one example at this point, an example that for us has a great deal of significance for our present task, of making Natural Therapy known to those who can be helped by it or to help others through it, the probability of our happening to be conversing in any ordinary situation with someone who has the kinds of problems for which the therapy was designed is one in three, or 33%. If inborn conditionability is normally distributed in the population as are similar natural characteristics, then only one-third of the population are predisposed to have significant problems. Of this group only the grandiose ones among them are likely to have such problems, so the expectation of an individual's being interested in the therapy is more realistically hardly as much as 15%. Such knowledge, besides preventing us from misjudging the behavior of others, assists us to know our audience and tailor our attempts to reach them. As those in the field of communication know, if you can't define your audience, you don't have one.

FEEDBACK FROM RADIO PROGRAMS

Like others who advocate a new approach to living, we have now and then been interviewed on radio talk shows, though not by the most well-known ones. The result of one of these interviews was that we were invited to present a weekly one-half hour program on a non-commercial radio station in a large Midwestern city. At this writing we have just completed our twentieth such program, and have decided to stop to assess the results of this kind of exposure for the therapy.

Two of our students in the social and behavioral sciences assisted us in the preparation and delivery of these programs, a project in which we had to more articulately and precisely define Natural Therapy concepts, and also to apply the therapy to a wider variety of specific problems than ever.

After devoting the first six programs to an explanation of the fundamentals of Natural Therapy, we applied the therapy to the following problems areas. Our comments about each are designed to furnish only brief indicators of how Natural Therapy principles apply to them.

Guilt and Infer- Natural Therapy holds that normal
iority Feelings   guilt presents no significant prob-
                  lem, while "neurotic guilt" (inability to forgive one's self) does and is due to grandiosity. Neurotic guilt is often "free-floating." Inferiority feelings result from fear of failure, which one's grandiosity cannot tolerate.

Fears and   When the object of fear is specific
Phobias   and known, it presents no signifi-

cant problem. Anxiety, especially of the "free-floating" variety, is a significant problem due to overconcern about self. Phobias related to a specific object are due to some specific severe conditioning and are rather easily overcome through reconditioning such as behavior modification. "Free-floating" phobic reactions are similar to "free-floating" anxiety, with the same cause and cure.

Depression   Principally two basic types are defined on the basis of their origin. The functionally-derived kind are due to grandiosity. The physically-derived kind are made worse by grandiosity.

Suicidal   About 20% of individuals with such
Feelings   feelings have some physical malfunction related to them. If anyone is worried about having this variety, he doesn't have it. The functionally-derived kind are due to grandiosity, and attempted suicide by those that have them is regarded as the ultimate ego trip, by which they unconsciously are attempting to have the last word, even if it kills them.

Self-Love   Non-grandiose individuals are not
Self-Hate   concerned about this. To love self, one must be lovable. One becomes lovable through Natural Therapy, illustrated also by Dr. Selye's advice: "Earn your neighbor's love."

Major Social   Since many have significant prob-
Problems   lems related to social problems, we apply Natural Therapy to them, both in a general as well as in a specific way. Generally we show that the therapy is highly relevant whether one views social problems from the point of view of the victim, as was usually done in the past, or from the newer structure-function point of view. The latter views the changing of the

structure and/or its function as the antidote, but it has become quite obvious that this is very difficult to do. Natural Therapy suggests that the grandiosity of the power-elite, who maintain dysfunction in the social structure for their own self-interest, be modified through the application of Natural Therapy principles. The problems of the victims of this dysfunction can be alleviated as illustrated in the following personal problems that are also major social problems.

Mental Disorders   Natural Therapy agrees largely with those who hold that mental illness is a myth. If a disorder in this area is physically induced, as we believe such manifestations as so-called manic-depression and schizophrenia basically are, then it should be regarded and treated as a physical illness, thus removing much of the stigma presently attached to it. Sometimes grandiosity is added to such physical illnesses, exaggerating the symptoms. Mental disorders that are of functional origin are looked upon the same as so-called "neuroses," which are due to grandiosity, and include such significant problems as undue anger, paranoia, jealousy, and the common problems we have already described such as anxiety, inferiority, guilt, and phobias, which usually do not become major social problems.

Poverty and Ill-Health   While these are two distinct problems, we treat them together, because more often than not they are acquired through no known fault of the individuals who have them. While in some cases grandiosity may be an indirect cause of either or both (as in the case of an individual being poor, because he is too grandiose to take the kinds of jobs available, or another being in ill-health, because he is too grandiose to take recommended health measures), in those instances where the situation is beyond the control of the individual, it becomes a significant problem only if the individual refuses to accept it, the result of grandiosity.

Alcoholism and Drug Addiction — Both are regarded as addictions, and the result of grandiosity. Easily-conditioned grandiose individuals indulge to escape grandiosity-induced problems. Difficult-to-condition grandiose ones indulge as a result of a grandiosity-induced need for "kicks." The secret of the success of AA and similar treatment programs is their insistence on addicts making sacrifices to help other addicts.

Interpersonal Behavior Problems — Actually, Natural Therapy holds that all significant problems are problems in interpersonal relationships, including crime and delinquency. Then, of course, they are all the result of grandiosity. Much more is said about interpersonal relationshps later in this book, where Natural Therapy's views in this area are described at length.

Marriage and Family Problems — The many problems in this area are due to the factors we describe when we explain problems of interpersonal relationships referred to above. While again we want to refer you to our later treatment of that, it might satisfy any present curiosity if we add that the basic approach of Natural Therapy is that such problems, especially in marriage and the family, are due to a grandiosity-induced need for dependency.

Sex Problems — In addition to the interpersonal relationship problems that certainly are also found in the area of sex, much of the problem here is due to the vast ignorance that apparently exists about the basic sexual natures of the male and the female. In addition, however, wherever there are expectations regarding the way to perform sexually, it is grandiosity that is at the root of any functional problems.

Child-Rearing In this area Natural Therapy has important relevance to the more important matter of *preventing* significant problems. Parents may prevent their offspring from becoming grandiose, and thus help them to escape the development of significant problems in life.

Problems in all Life Stages In the concluding program we followed all subsequent life stages from adolescence to old age. The problems that are characteristic of each of them can always be traced to grandiosity and be coped with by modifying grandiosity.

The therapy for each of them is basically that which we outline in the final chapters of this book. We hope that this brief treatment of the application of the therapy to these problems, though our summary of 200 pages of script has to be totally inadequate, will give the reader additional insights into the therapy as it now exists. Complete information on these and other programs available on cassettes are obtainable from The Natural Therapy Foundation, 5 Greenleaf, Irvine, California 92714.

THE RECENT RESEARCH OF OTHERS

When we began to put our Natural Therapy together with biological determinism at its basis, we had the feeling that we were one of the few voices crying in the wilderness. We had maintained a close tie with the academic world of the social and behavioral sciences by part-time teaching at universities and colleges, and by the faithful reading of the journals from a number of the leading related professional societies in which we have held membership for many years, and it was quite evident that environmental determinism was in complete command, at least in American psychology and sociology. Little did we know that among a few prestigious academicians in these areas a revolt against environmental determinism was brewing. It came to our attention in 1975 when we used the newly-published textbook *Man in Society* written by Pierre L. van den Berghe as an auxiliary text in one of our sociology courses.

We don't know whether van den Berghe's gutsy book gave the necessary courage to others with ideas of a similar kind, but all of a sudden we began to come across a number of articles advocating sociobiology, which was a kind of emphasis on a great deal of the biological as determiners of human social behavior, employing a great amount of data from anthropology and evolution. For us it had reached its current zenith in a proclamation by Edward O. Wilson, a Harvard University entomologist and sociobiologist, reported recently in the *Los Angeles Times* (April 19, 1979), that "there is no longer any serious question from even the sharpest critics that a genetic basis for behavior has been found." He goes on to claim that there is a genetic basis for such personality traits as *introversion, extraversion, neurosis, schizophrenia, homosexuality* (italics ours), and sports ability. You can understand how much we welcomed these kinds of claims that related so specifically to some of the key principles of our therapy. But he also went on to claim that some genes also predispose to aggression, *sex, altruism,* and *religion* (italics ours), and you will better understand our interest in that in our discussion of religion and altruism in the following chapter.

It is also interesting that some in psychology have recently become interested in studying the so-called "invulnerables," those who are exposed to the environmental influences that are said by prevailing American psychology to cause behavior problems, but who do not develop them. We contacted those who were studying these "invulnerables" and they replied that they have not yet discovered why this happens. We would hazard the guess that they are looking for causes in the environment, and we don't believe they will find them there.

Whenever we ask the environmental determinists why one sibling behaves one way and his brother in the opposite way, even though they are subjected day in and day out to the same environment, the only explanation we get is that there must be some other factor, an environmental one, of course, that is intervening, but which is also unknown to them. And, when we persist, and ask them to suggest what this intervening variable might possibly be, we find it easy to shoot down what they suggest, so that finally they say that it must be accepted as an unknown, and apparently an unknowable one.

Think of the grandiosity that has to be involved in setting forth the likely causes of important behavior, when there are more exceptions to the rules they set than those who conform. And, even more amazing, when an intervening variable may be at work, which, they fail to add, must be the most important consideration in trying to determine causes, if, in effect, it is the intervening variable that also prevents the majority from displaying it. Of course, if it is admitted that the intervening variable is some biological influence, like inborn degree of conditionability, then their problem is solved.

Even our eye-doctor made a contribution that at least reaffirmed our biological determinism. When he asked us on our recent visit to his office what we were doing these days, and we told him about our Natural Therapy work, he quickly added: "It's about time you behavioral scientists learned what we physicians have always known, that, to be free of problems, choose your parents wisely. It's drilled into us every day when we have to treat son, father, and grandfather of the same family."

We don't have space to include additional evidence for much of what Natural Therapy stands for from the research of others. Much of it is also coming from the so-called biosociologists, who are similarly interested in promoting the biological basis of social behavior but without the evolutionary approach, from psychobiologists, and a great variety of other sources, which often furnish newspapers with headlines like the following that we have seen:

"Cheating Husband? Blame It On Genes."
"Genes *Ueber Alles.*"
"Heredity Seen As A Factor In Anxiety."
"The Biological Need For High Stimulation."
"Whatever Parents Do, Some Children Are Born
   To Be Different."
"Being A Teacher Is In The Genes."

OUR OWN FURTHER RESEARCH

We've already referred to the fact that one of the most important discoveries we have made subsequent to the first putting together of the therapy is the discovery of the part that compulsions or have-tos play, both in the development of significant problems as well as in preventing many from putting into practice the things they must do to solve those problems. This discovery was very fruitful in many different ways in the whole area of solving significant problems as well as preventing them in the first place.

It led us, together with one of our classes, to develop what we call our Have-To Inventory, designed to measure the presence and the degree of the have-tos that problem people have. Originally composed to be a helpful tool for counselors to help them determine their clients' have-tos and also to convince clients of their grandiosity, if they did not want to admit it, as they sometimes did not, it was to be a companion to another tool of the counselor, the Eysenck Personality Inventory, which measured especially the client's inborn degree of conditionability. With these two objective and proven tests, a counselor could in about 20 minutes determine what part the two key components of the Natural Therapy system play in the client's problem.

And we ourself used them very successfully for this purpose on a number of occasions. After the HTI was completed, we had to norm the scores.

At this point we got the brilliant idea of making up an interview schedule composed of three parts: our HTI, an EII (Extravision-Introversion Inventory), and an inventory that included a number of correlates having to do with the background of the respondent. It was our idea through this schedule not only to determine the scores for differing age and sex groups, but also to see how the following variables we were measuring correlated with each other: the have-to score, the conditionability score, age, sex, marital status, education, church membershp, having a serious problem, self-designation regarding extraversion-introversion, extraversion-introversion of parents and siblings, leadership-followership self-designation, self-rating of intelligence and of being religious, and self-designation of degree of emotionality and of altruism. You can see from this description that, in addition to its use in establishing norms for the HTI scores, this information is very helpful in validating the entire theoretical system that undergirds Natural Therapy and in suggesting additional improvement and application of the therapy.

At this writing we have sampled the entries in about 500 completed schedules presently available to us, and have received more than sufficient evidence from them thus far to demonstrate that the theoretical basis of the Natural Therapy system is so sound, that we have decided that it is not necessary to include our HTI in an Appendix of this book, as we earlier had planned, for self-administration by the reader.

Through this survey we have been assured that, when an individual has a significant problem, one which is affecting almost every area of his life, then that individual is grandiose and has strong have-tos. When an individual has a significant problem in only one area of his life, and which does not importantly impair his ability to function adequately in other areas, then it is not the typical problem for which Natural Therapy is indicated, and it is not due to grandiosity and its inherent compulsions. Then there is no need to objectively measure have-tos.

An interesting discovery that resulted from this same survey was that respondents did not do very well in correctly designating their own degree of extraversion-introversion, and this had led us to consider the inclusion of a self-administered inventory to measure also that objectively. But when other parts of the survey confirmed our claim that easy-to-condition grandiose people have significant problems mainly of the emotional variety, and the difficult-to-condition grandiose mainly of the behavioral type, we concluded here also that it was not necessary to include an inventory to measure degree of conditionability. In a face-to-face counseling situation, however, we invariably use our HTI and the EPI to quickly determine the degree of involvement of these two key components.

Hopefully, by the time that we are ready to publish our projected *Readings in Natural Therapy* volume, we will have analyzed more completely the data from the aforementioned survey, and will include a chapter on the findings in that forthcoming book.

This chapter would not be complete without at least a brief mention of another important support for our approach that has come from an entirely unexpected area. We have cited, though not described at length, some important support for biological determinism that has come recently from behavioral and related sciences. Now, out of the blue, we have just learned of a Kohutian (Heinz Kohut, University of Chicago psychiatrist) movement in psychoanalysis that is claiming that narcissism (defined as "apparent self-love and grandiosity") is the leading illness of our time. While we are in some disagreement with Kohut's description of its origin and cure, we welcome this recognition of the importance of grandiosity in significant problems.

The brief summary in this chapter of additional discoveries about Natural Therapy, since its first appearance, has pointed out not only some important confirmation of the basic theory involved, but, even more importantly, the need to integrate such information into a much-improved and more helpful Natural Therapy. This we have tried to do in the remainder of this book.

chapter **4**

Additional Insights
From Religion

WE AMPLIFY OUR VIEWS

Our original intention in writing a second book about Natural Therapy was to give religion the most prominent place. In our first draft of the manuscript we not only devoted 104 pages to it, but we openly stated in the manuscript that it was our opinion that the basic principles of Biblical Christianity not only agreed with the principles that undergirded Natural Therapy, but that to approach the therapy from that direction was by far the best way to implement it. We went so far as to frequently refer to the therapy as God's Therapy and Scriptural Therapy.

We had been led to this kind of promotion of Biblical Christianity in connection with our therapy because of the discoveries we had made subsequent to the first appearnce of our original book. As we have previously indicated, we had made an exhaustive research into scientific psychology and discovered what genuine experimental psychology had found, and it became the basis of the underlying principles for our therapy.

We have also stated that much of this sounded strangely familiar, and seemed to be proving much of what some Scripture passages were saying, passages that had always seemed to us to be saying more than what our church thought they were saying. So we decided that our first great need was to research Scripture as thoroughly as possible, especially after our first book came out.

The religious part of our first book reflected essentially what our own church body had been teaching in areas that seemed to us to relate to Natural Therapy. There we made an initial attempt to fit scientific psychology and our church's teaching together, and they seemed to coincide remarkably well. In fact, even though our church body had recently been on an extended heresy hunt, we were very much pleased that the professionals in our denomination voiced no appreciable opposition to the doctrinal content of our first book. And we were especially pleased by the enthusiastic reception of it by the laity.

Our subsequent research into Scripture resulted in so many more remarkable confirmations of the therapy that, in our earlier manuscript for this second book, we devoted about one-third of it to that. Eventually, however, we were led to see its remarkable relevance to *all* major religions, and it is this that we summarize in this chapter. *Do keep in mind throughout that the therapy is not designed for the acquiring of spiritual gifts such as faith, forgiveness, and eternal life, though it has some relevance to their preservation wherever they are threatened in the presence of significant earthly problems.*

RELIGION TEACHES A BIOLOGICAL DETERMINISM

Paradoxically, while the major religions and their adherents operate almost invariably on the basis of an environmental determinist approach to human behavior, their official teachings admit only a predominant biological determinist view. Every major religion believes that God, or whatever name they use for the Supreme Being, is the Lord and Ruler of the Universe, and that God is ruling it in the interest of the spiritual and temporal survival and progress of His creation. Moreover in no major religion are His creatures, especially human beings, exempted from being His agents in carrying out His government and providence of the universe. In fact, each one of them is to have as his prime purpose in life the duty as well as privilege to glorify God, which can in essence be done only by using himself primarily for the spiritual and temporal welfare of all of God's creation, especially humankind.

These truths can be demonstrated by the specific teachings of each of these religions, and, of course, can also be deduced without them. Biblical Christianity is certainly an outstanding example of this, and we need not go into detail to demonstrate it, as we did originally in our earlier manuscript for this book.

If, in the light of what has just been pointed out, any religion teaches an *environmental* determinism in human behavior, that is, if it teaches that human behavior is principally influenced by external conditioning, then that religion has literally dethroned God as Lord and Ruler of the Universe. For, if God has indeed decided principally to use humankind to carry out His government and providence of the universe (and it is quite evident that He has, as we can see also from what makes for survival and progress of the universe), and if His government and providence cannot fail (as is also quite evident at least thus far in a universe that has both survived and progressed despite many great obstacles), then certainly it has to be due principally to the fact that He has created human beings with the necessary ability to act in this respect according to His will for the universe, and has insured that no external conditioning agent could ever condition such qualities *out,* significantly modify them, or condition *in* any qualities that might significantly oppose them.

It is obvious to us that the Creator has insured that His will in this be carried out by His placing such qualities into the genes and chromosomes of human beings. That is why we say that religion, as we usually find it, basically teaches a biological determinism.

Now some may argue that, with all the advances in genetic engineering, it could be possible to change God's will in this respect. But again, on the basis of Natural Therapy principles, whenever God's will has to do with important matters, He builds in controls to make certain that at least a sufficient number of individuals will act in accordance with His will, so that eventually it is carried out. One of such controls is that individuals would have significant problems if they did not act in accordance with His design for them, and enough would on that account return to behavior that would again coincide with God's basic will for them. Thus, in genetic engineering, while it might eventually prove a useful gift of God to engineer out undesirable qualities, one could be certain that trying to change an obvious design of an individual for the part that he needs to play in the progress and preservation of the universe would be beset with significant problems for humankind.

The reader can see in this what a religious view of significant problems can do to confirm biological determinism, one of the important truths upon which our therapy rests. In view of all this it is difficult to understand why religious people, especially when trying to solve significant problems, try to extricate themselves from them through ways that are basically environmental-deterministic. For example, they often seek help from self-help books or from counselors that use those kinds of approaches.

By the same token, it is also hard to comprehend why pastors and churches and church denominations base their programs of worship, counseling, education, evangelism, and stewardship — the key areas of their mission — on approaches that are based on environmental-determinist considerations, even while their basic doctrines proclaim the very opposite.

It is our educated opinion that, just as prevailing American therapy has a very sorry record of success with significant problems, practically everywhere the key congregational programs are in sorry shape for the same reasons. In contrast, we also know of a few congregations which are making rudimentary attempts to do the opposite and are highly successful.

This also has implications for religious people with significant problems who are interested in using Natural Therapy. We had good intentions in including a lengthy chapter on religion in our first book. They had to do with helping the religious person to be more zealous in putting the basic principles and techniques of the therapy into practice. But evidently for many, it succeeded mostly in confirming the truth of their religious convictions, and, though they tried the techniques, they did it with overtones of the magical way in which they also employed their religion. We have a great deal more to say about that in a later section.

Taking their cue from what we've just stated, readers, aware now of their religion's confirmation of biological determinism in human behavior, should find it easier to accept the principles and techniques of Natural Therapy, and to put them into practice more zealously if they desire to use it for any significant problem besetting their life.

RELIGIOUS PEOPLE ARE EASILY CONDITIONED

We have in a previous chapter indicated the confirmation of our contention, made already in our first book, that religious people are invariably of the introverted or, better, easily-conditioned type. Some people are born religious, as also the Harvard professor mentioned earlier has insisted on the basis of all the evidence for it. When religious people, especially pastors, hear this, they are often shocked. Some follow it up with: "So we're just robots, are we?"

We can understand these kinds of reactions, for religious people often feel that they have come consciously to believe in their religion, or God Himself planted their faith in them, or, in any case, they aren't robots, for, in fact, it is also because of their religion that they have greater control of their lives than those who are not religious.

In our first book we devoted one section to try to show how the Scriptures teach an inborn conditionability that varies with individuals. While we could add further evidence from Scripture here, we would rather devote our treatment of it here to try to meet the objections that some religious people have to it.

Inborn easy-conditionability need not make any religious person or anyone else a robot. Remember that Natural Therapy holds that behavior is determined by one's biology only to about 80 or 85% (we get those percentages from experiments designed to try to modify biological characteristics through manipulation by environmental agents). Perhaps it is easier to understand it if it is expressed in this way: our biological makeup determines the way we will act in certain kinds of situations, while the environment (or the conditioning agent) provides the opportunity to act and also offers different choices of the manner in which such action can be carried out. (In all this, though, it must be kept in mind that the biological can compel us to act even when the environment is not providing any opportunity to do so.)

For example, suppose your pastor asks you to take over his Sunday Bible Class on a day when he had to be away. You may not be grandiose, but, because you are easily-conditioned, you take his request seriously. That doesn't mean that you will agree to his request; you have previously agreed to attend your nephew's confirmation that Sunday at another location, and you do not want to disappoint him. Or you may feel that you honestly could not do an adequate job of this important assignment. Or you may be able to get some other competent person to teach the class. In other words, your type of conditionability leads you to take the whole matter seriously, which forces you to take into account all the concerns inherent in the situation. Yet, you do have a choice in what you finally will do in the matter, which finally may eventuate in many different forms that your response may take. In that sense you would not be acting like a robot. The final form of action can very well satisfy also your own interests in the matter.

Thus the religious person does not need to become upset by the finding that religious people are invariably of the easily-conditioned type, and were born that way. If, as many religious people believe, it is God alone Who creates a faith in Him in the hearts of the believers, what would be wrong with Him making it all easier and more natural by creating some of them as people who are more receptive to religion because of inborn seriousness? Besides, they would also later, as His followers, resist less the divinely-inspired impulse to do His will.

And anyway, as someone has also said, to whom would they proclaim the good news of their faith, if all were the same as they and had faith already? These, of course, are not really appropriate questions, but there is a question that does have relevance: Does it not seem unfair of the Creator to create some individuals who are apparently more predisposed to become religious?

Our answer to that has been that certainly God could overcome any obstacle to enable an individual to come to faith, and no doubt He does. While it's true that you won't find many difficult-to-condition individuals in the organized church (and when you do find them there, it is often due to the fact that they have either been born into the church, or some spouse or friend has pressured them into joining, or they may even have some ulterior reasons for their membership), there no doubt are many such persons outside the organized church who are religious. Psychologist Samenow, whose work confirms much of Natural Therapy, has found that even the most hardened criminal, among the so-called criminally-insane, often indicated a great respect for God and religion.

In the final analysis, the question about why God

created some more predisposed to religion than others is similar to the question that bothers many Christians: Can anyone be saved if he does not believe in Christ, even though he apparently had no opportunity even to hear about Him? The answer we always gave was the only one we felt that the Scriptures themselves give: any failure to come to such faith will be judged on the basis of the opportunities he had to acquire it. Certainly one's biological equipment is also involved with degree of opportunity.

We hope we've laid to rest some of the concerns that religious people may have about inborn degree of conditionability. But it's imperative that we recognize the importance of the kind of conditionability we have, so that we will be more zealous in pursuing the proper use of it in Natural Therapy, remembering that the most important aspect of that kind of conditionability is that it makes us more concerned individuals. And that, in turn, should lead us to use that concern primarily to help humankind to survive and progress spiritually and temporally. Incidentally, the concept here of survival has special meaning for religious people. In fact, it ought to be somewhat mind-boggling in view of the fact that, in their kind of belief, such survival can reach eternal proportions under heavenly conditions. To use one's self, then, to have an important part in helping others to that kind of survival . . . (is there anything left to add?).

RELIGION RECOGNIZES GRANDIOSITY

In the preceding section we gave some attention to some religious aspects of inborn conditionability, one of the key components of the Natural Therapy system. Here we take a look at some of the important implications for religious people of the other key component — grandiosity.

One might expect that religious people especially are prone to develop grandiosity, for all the ingredients are there that can make people grandiose. We've already mentioned the obvious easy-conditionability that characterizes religious individuals. Their parents most likely were also religious, and thus highly concerned and overprotective regarding the welfare and security of their children. In Scripture children are described as a special gift of God. When brought to church and church school at an early age, such children learn that they are children of God, heirs of heaven, watched over by angels. What easily-conditioned child could escape grandiosity under the influence of all that?

One would normally expect that, with all of religion's assurances of the status of God's children in the eyes of God — people made in God's image, chosen of God, royal priests, special objects of God's concern, and the like — religious people would be the last ones to display any great fear, any disabling feelings of inferiority, any unresolved feelings of guilt, any feelings of being unloved. Yet it is common knowledge, especially among counselors, that religious people usually display more of these kinds of significant problems than those who are not religious. The latter are the ones that display a much greater amount of *behavior* problems than religious people. This, of course, is what we can expect from those that are essentially difficult-to-condition, as those uninterested in religion usually are.

So we should not be surprised to discover so many significant emotional-type problems among religious people. Nor should we be surprised to find a great incidence of such problems also and especially among pastors, for, as we have indicated already in an earlier chapter, pastors have generally been found to be even more grandiose than many lay members. It is not surprising, then, in the present age, aptly described as the "me" generation, when grandiosity is more rampant than ever before, to our knowledge, that one hears fewer and fewer sermons on sin and hell and damnation, but more and more sermons on what great people we are because we are children of God, and so we must love ourselves, quit downgrading ourselves, believe in our own brilliance as a famous TV preacher recently put it, etc. One gets the feeling that such preachers are really talking to themselves, and, if they are, we know the reason why.

One can understand that kind of approach from some of the newer psychologically-oriented churches that are springing up here and there these days, but to hear that from churches, that confess the Scriptures as the basis of their teaching, is almost unbelievable. Where in the Scriptures does it say that our significant problems are due to our poor self-image, our feelings of inferiority? Nowhere.

But there are a large number of passages that tells us that it is our pride that causes our problems and can even destroy us. Unfortunately, the word pride today often has a good meaning, but that is not the way that Scripture means it. A few of the newer English translations, like Phillips and the New English Bible, use the more accurate word "arrogance," which, as you can see, has more the flavor of the grandiosity that, Natural Therapy holds, is at the bottom of our feelings of fear, inferiority, guilt, etc.

Our emphasis here on religion's confirmation of the direct source of significant problems in the grandiosity that even, and quite often, religious people especially have, should certainly induce them to use Natural Therapy zealously as God's own remedy for it, as we show especially in the ensuing section.

NATURAL THERAPY AS GOD'S OR
SCRIPTURAL THERAPY

We pointed out already in our first book that the major religions of the world teach that the Golden Rule is an important, if not the most important, part of their religion. The Golden Rule, as most people know, commands us to "do unto others as we would have others do unto us." And, at first thought, it sounds quite simple, innocent, innocuous, and rather easy to carry out. Some might look at it with a little alarm at the thought of what it could permit and still be observed. This may give you an inkling of how the real requirement of the Golden Rule can easily be overlooked or misinterpreted.

Almost everyone views the Golden Rule as a command to give equal treatment to others, treatment that matches that which we give to ourselves. But that is not what the Rule says; it commands us to give to others the same treatment that we *want* them to give to us. And if we are honest, we will admit that we *want, desire, wish* that others would place our interests ahead of their own. Our normal interest in self-preservation impels us to have that kind of want, desire, and wish for ourselves. If we are grandiose, with more than the minimal amount of self-interest necessary for self-preservation, such want, desire, and wish for ourselves is also highly compulsive.

That kind of want, desire, and wish, says the Golden Rule, should characterize our treatment of others. In other words, it is plainly stating that, in our treatment of others, we should place their interests *ahead* of our own. And by this time we should have no trouble identifying this requirement as central in Natural Therapy. Thus also this religious consideration can add immeasurably to the reliability and validity of the therapy, and indicate again that, like religion, it has stood the test of time. That alone should make religious people more zealous to practice it, especially for significant problems.

While we arrived at the central idea in Natural Therapy, which is to use our natural qualities primarily for humankind, through the idea in all major religions that God is the Ruler and Preserver and Provider of the universe, and that He uses humans as His agents to carry out His government and providence, we are particularly pleased that teachings like the Golden Rule actually spell out that central idea. In fact, in Biblical Christianity, there are a number of additional passages that do the same.

Now it is quite evident that few religious persons even try to observe the erroneous view of the Golden Rule, that is, to try to give others *equal* treatment. And even fewer try to give others *priority,* as the Rule really implies, and which even some additional passages clearly confirm. But it surprises almost every Biblical Christian, for example, and a surprisingly large number of their pastors, that there are a number of clear New Testament passages that command Christians to give 100% and *exclusive* attention to the interests of others. Religious people very seldom hear about those passages, and we're sure that they have not ever heard a sermon on any of them. In fact, almost all modern translations do not correctly translate some of them, apparently because their requirement is hardly acceptable, even to those who profess to believe in the verbal infallibility of Scripture. Those passages say, in effect: Use your natural qualities completely and exclusively for the welfare of others.

What should the Biblical Christian do about such demands? Remember that in Natural Therapy, we do not suggest that natural qualities be used *exclusively* for others. We use the word *primarily.* And we do so because we feel that in our day individuals find it more difficult to deal with significant problems than those in Biblical times, and we did not want to discourage people by advocating a therapy that would be practically impossible to carry out.

At the same time we wish to acknowledge the superiority of the Biblical approach and demand, because it is psychologically much superior. While no one can ever fully and exclusively use himself for others, by demanding the ultimate of us, it keeps us striving, even though we can never reach that ultimate goal. Most of our humanly-devised therapies today require us to only do the best we can, and perhaps that is an important reason why they are also so ineffective.

RELIGION VIEWS ALTRUISM

We would suggest that what we state here is one of the most important considerations in Natural Therapy, and we will admit that our original presentation in our first book was thoroughly inadequate in this area. Though we did state that our natural qualities were given "partly for the individual's own survival and general well-being," we followed that by adding that they were given "primarily for the survival and welfare of others."

We should have amplified that statement, so that it would not be misunderstood. Some took that statement, and even the whole therapy approach, to mean that we need to become as unselfish as possible if we are to get the desired result from the therapy, despite the fact that there were very many other statements in the book that indicated that those who practice giving of themselves for others would get more in return for themselves.

And, paradoxically, it was some religious people especially who appeared to take exception to that view and openly admitted to us that they feel reluctant to use the therapy, knowing that they were doing so because of the large rewards that they would receive when they did.

These two kinds of opposite reactions led us to do a great deal of research into the whole area of altruism, which has always been a controversial concept. We ourself had had trouble in the past trying to trap it, and, after our recent further research into it, we came away wondering why anyone in religion could advocate and try to implement it properly in such a simple way as they evidently try to do. In our recollection of our seminary studies, we don't recall that the concept ever came up for special consideration.

Of course, with the Lutheran basic emphasis on being saved alone by faith and without good works, one can understand that the idea of altruism would be considerably neglected, for one had to avoid any semblance of work-righteousness at all costs. We recall with great amusement our great concerns about the reaction of fellow-pastors in our church body when, in a Reformation Sunday service at our historic Trinity Church in Los Angeles about ten years ago, we dared to preach a sermon on "Faith Without

Works Is Dead.''

A Reformation service traditionally was expected to de-emphasize works. And our concern mounted when we learned after the service from the president of the congregation, that great churchman Dr. Shau Wa Chan, that there was in attendance that day a very distinguished gentleman who took copious notes during the sermon. That gentleman was the well-known Dan Thrapp, the religion editor of the *Los Angeles Times,* and you can imagine the heights that our concerns finally reached when, in the next morning's issue of that popular newspaper, there appeared a rather lengthy summary of that sermon.

The absence of any adverse response to that sermon might indicate that some of our fellow-pastors were practicing altruism, or that, like us at the time, they evidently had that inner gut-feeling that good works were being sadly overlooked in our church body. And, in this connection, we ought to state that perhaps our persistent apparent overemphasis on justification without works in our churches was no doubt partly due to the common experience of pastors that, no matter how clearly they taught Luther's Reformation theme — faith without works, when they asked their members how they hoped to be saved, the quick reply of too many of them would invariably be: ''By being good.'' And that, of course, would include doing good for others.

It is interesting in this connection to recall something that we mentioned earlier, that a number of current researchers, particularly sociobiologists like Edward Wilson of Harvard, have insisted that altruism is basically biologically-derived behavior. Even before them, a number of social psychologists had included the phenomenon of ''mutual-aid'' in the list of basic human needs and drives.

All this has kind of added up for us a great deal of evidence for our idea of inborn conditionability, and particularly here the important part that it may play in producing altruistic behavior. The latter would indicate to us that it had to be the easily-conditioned type individual's behavior that led Wilson, Kropotkin, and their kind to their conclusions. These are also the types that are commonly found in churches. Is it any wonder that they should have problems in de-emphasizing the importance of good works in one area of expected religious behavior?

Some might counter with the question: Why then do so many fail to do good works when their church expects and even commands them to? The answer is not only easy, but it also confirms another important principle of Natural Therapy: they are grandiose.

These insights that we already had acquired into altruistic behavior, as a result of our experiences with religious people, were greatly increased through our extensive research of what sociologists, psychologists, and philosophers had found about it. Though we had years earlier taken some interest in their views about altruism, and remembered that our conclusion had been that there seemed to be no general agreement about its definition or even its possibility, we now discovered that, with perhaps only one exception, those who had studied altruism appeared to be agreed that all altruism is basically selfish, no matter how one defines it. In other words, there really can be no behavior that has as its dominant feature an interest in helping another. And so, except for some philosophers, whose domain anyway is basically to determine, on the basis of reason, whether any conceivable or observable phenomenon is possible, the concept of altruism has been largely abandoned, also by behavioral scientists, and even by theologians, as not viable, if not impossible.

The only exception, to our knowledge, among earlier students of altruism, was Pitirim Sorokin, in many ways the peerless sociologist, who was highly interested in social problems, and was finally forced to conclude that only altruism could eliminate them. He did a good deal of research in altruism, and did come up with the only appreciable scientific evidence for its utility up to that time, and he wrote up his findings in several books, which, even though they make for interesting reading especially for today, have been largely ignored. The more recent exceptions to those who have abandoned the study of altruism are, of course, the sociobiologists.

Sociobiologists, while proceeding from evolutionary considerations, are saying much the same that biosociologists are saying these days, who proceed from nonevolutionary bases, as does also the present author, who might be classified also as one of them. In either or both instances, the conclusions of both of them, regarding the biological sources of human behavior, are given additional support from the principles we advance in Natural Therapy.

While the additional evidences referred to above can proceed from our therapy's claims about inborn conditionability, perhaps our attempts to integrate the therapy with the widespread religious confirmation of it, in the teachings of the major religions, lends support of the kind they have not yet investigated. We know that such evidence, simply because it has something to do with God, often is of little interest to sociologists and biologists. Of course, it would be highly unscientific of them not to be interested in religiosity, that is, the behavior of religious people as such. In addition, a consideration of a certain teaching of religion, as viewed from the acceptance or rejection of it by its adherents, is an important aspect of religiosity that relates importantly to the scientific investigation of behavioral phenomena. Such an investigation could not leave out the important variable of the human perception of some religious doctrine.

Relating this to altruistic behavior, Natural Therapy holds that religion generally has to agree with the idea of a biological source of such behavior. In our view, when we speak of the biological determinism of altruistic behavior, we mean the determination to practice it or not to practice it, which differs in individuals. We've already indicated how religious people, by nature generally easily-conditioned, apparently know the importance of altruistic behavior, but so many of them do not practice it because of grandiosity.

This idea may seem to be contrary to the teaching, generally found among Biblically-oriented Christians especially, that all humans by nature know the Moral Law, which basically enjoins them to behave altruistically. That doctrine comes from St. Paul's assertion in Romans 2 that apparently *some,* who were not Jews and didn't know the Mosaic Law, still acted in accordance with it. Unfortunately, many English translations lead us to believe that *all* non-Jews displayed such conformity, which the original text does not say. If it did, then it would be in contradiction to what anthropologists have consistently found — that behavior, even in the most-important areas of the Moral Law, is far from universally consistent, both intraculturally and interculturally.

The original, of course, is correct — some people behave altruistically, even and often without specific directions, rather spontaneously. These, of course, in Natural Therapy's view, would be the non-grandiose easily-conditioned ones. Is this not also what St. Paul means when he adds later that this shows that the Law is written in their hearts? And doesn't this also solve the ongoing controversy among Bible-believing Christians about whether a believer still needs God's Law, as some Scripture passages seem to deny? The obvious implication is that, if one is truly Christian, he will "instinctively"(?) know what is correct behavior in any situation and act accordingly.

If that is true, how does one explain the fact that sometimes an apparently true Christian will behave contrary to God's Law? Didn't even Paul confess that he did not always do what was good, even though he wanted to? Such considerations have led some to establish a Third Use of the Law, which is to remind Christians what are truly good works in God's sight.

Natural Therapy has a solution to the dilemma that seems to be involved in this controversy. It is simply again that Christians, that is, those that believe in Christ as their Savior and even as Lord, can and do develop grandiosity, just as they can and do develop arthritis, and this so distorts any situation for them, that they choose to behave in a certain manner in that situation which appears to them, especially at the time, to be acceptable Christian behavior.

If that means also that we think St. Paul could have been grandiose, that is correct. It should not take any reader of his Letters very long to see it. How else could you describe anyone who sometimes wrote something to this effect: "This is what God has to say about this, but here's what I say about it . . ."? One could cite a hundred more examples of his apparent grandiosity.

In sum, religion, while it teaches the importance of altruistic behavior, both because it indicates the involvement of the biological, as well as the need for it, in the design for the survival and progress of humankind, also explains why some practice it and others do not.

RELIGION HELPS US UNDERSTAND CONSCIENCE

While conscience, no matter how it has been defined, evidently plays an important part in human behavior, and especially also some behavior problems, it appears to be seldom used in therapy. Clergymen perhaps are about the only ones known to use it, or to try to use it, to influence human behavior. We remember a friend of ours once writing and delivering a paper titled: "Conscience, the Pastor's Ally." The title should already tell you something about the approach. It is our opinion that, due to a gross misunderstanding of what conscience really is and how it operates, it has not been used, as it could be, in therapy.

Our original concept of conscience was highly influenced by the rather simplistic approach to it that has characterized many religions. Behavioral scientists haven't done much better. Both groups have brought about much of the confusion themselves, because they have been unable to separate conscience from that which prompts it to go into action.

Actually the word conscience literally means "knowledge with" or "knowing with." Generally the word appears to connote that conscience is basically a comparison of one thing with another, or, more specifically, a judgment that is made of what an individual has thought, said, or done with what he knows he should have thought, said, or done. Conscience is generally thought of as that which goes into action to remind us when we have acted in any way against some internalized code of behavior.

Many have confused conscience with the code of behavior itself, which would considerably limit its function, in our opinion. We think it is safe to say that conscience is an inborn mechanism that goes into action whenever we think, say, or do anything, either to impart to us a good feeling, if it is in accord with how we feel about it ourselves, or to set in motion a bad feeling about it, if it is not in accord with what we feel about it ourselves.

It is evident from this view of conscience that we do not believe that this mechanism reacts to what we have been taught, but only to how we *feel* about what we have been taught, or, more technically, how much we have internalized of what we have been taught, our feelings about it being that which directly decides what we internalize. In turn, however, the nature of those feelings, whether approving, disapproving, or even just neutral, are indirectly determined by our inborn degree of conditionability.

However, if we become grandiose, then our feelings about anything we have been taught are distorted, so that the code of behavior that we internalize will be modified by the amount of that distortion, and we will have significant problems if we behave accordingly, as we are likely to do.

Now we begin to understand why the simplistic advice often given, like "let your conscience be your guide," can be quite inadequate. We also find it hard to understand the advice of some theologians who tell us that we must always obey our consciences, or that we should not sin against our conscience even when it is an erring one, although we never quite fully understood what was meant by the term erring conscience. Actually, with our view of conscience as simply an inborn mechanism that goes into action to approve or disapprove our behavior, to speak of obeying that or disobeying it makes no sense.

What they evidently mean, and what some passages in Scripture apparently do say, is that we should not go against the feelings we have about any behavior about which we have some good feelings of approval. This makes good sense, and it certainly is in accord with what we said before about those who are true believers — that they do not need any Law.

But it is also true, that we could have incorrect feelings about the rightness or wrongness of a certain type of behavior — what theologians erroneously call an erring conscience — something that can result from grandiosity, as we also explained earlier. But we should act in accordance with that wrong feeling anyway, even the Scripture assures the believer.

Does that make sense psychologically, or especially in terms of Natural Therapy? In one sense, that is an irrelevant question, because the individual involved does not know that his feelings are wrong in this matter, and would proceed to act accordingly, as his feelings indicated. What, then, is the purpose of saying that one should obey one's feelings about any behavior, contemplated or already completed?

Because in that way the individual would be learning to do the second important action that Natural Therapy advises if one wants to avoid or overcome significant problems in one's life, or, to put it positively, to be and to do what one was intended to be or to do to fulfill God's good and gracious will for the welfare of humankind.

If an individual has correct feelings about a certain behavior, then by indulging in it he is reinforcing both his thinking and acting habits that make for the fulfillment of his proper role in life. If his feelings are wrong about a certain behavior, the significant problems that ensue will force him to try to determine where he is wrong, and lead him hopefully to the kind of therapy, like Natural Therapy, that can help him see his grandiosity and deal properly with it. In either case, by obeying his feelings (not his conscience), any individual can learn to fulfill his proper mission in life.

It is no accident that many successful therapists, and even pastors, who often advise those whom they counsel to follow their feelings in making decisions, usually are helping them to make correct decisions. Not that such decisions are right in the sense that they always bring nothing but good, but in the sense that, if they are wrong, they can be led not only to see that they generally have wrong feelings about things, but also to discover why they have distorted feelings (grandiosity), and then to take steps to control it.

As an adviser to pastors in some of our capacities in church work, we have often been consulted by other pastors about the decision they had to make about a call, a position offered to them by a congregation or church body. While we usually helped them to weigh, in a more objective way than they usually could because they were more emotionally involved, the pros and cons, we always ended up by saying that they should finally make up their minds on the basis of how they really felt about the call, which they usually did. In almost every case, the decisions made on that basis apparently turned out well for them. In the few cases, where at first it seemed that they had made the wrong decision, in the long run it proved to be the correct one in retrospect.

It is to be understood, however, when Natural Therapy

advocates that we act on the basis of esoteric feelings, it does not mean this as a license to choose just any type of behavior. There are, certainly, some types of behavior that could be chosen that would bring significant and unnecessary harm to some individuals involved. The infinite variety of situations and choices of possible behavior in them make it quite impossible to be very specific in setting up criteria for guidance in this area. Perhaps the most that could be said is that the decision, about how far we should go in following our feelings, should be based generally upon what form of behavior, in the direction we feel we must proceed, will prove the least harmful to the least number of people who might be importantly affected by it.

We have arrived at this kind of solution, to an important consideration in implementing Natural Therapy on the basis of what we have always advised, when the therapy is to be implemented when other people are involved. Church people sometimes ask how far they can go in trying to change something that is going on in their congregation, and bringing harm to it, in their opinion at least. The very sensitive aspect of this kind of situation is that, in the process, some individuals in the congregation have to be opposed, and some unpleasant situations result.

We have always advised that generally one should proceed, or decide not to proceed, on the basis of the greatest good for the greatest number of those in the congregation that would result on the basis of the action taken. It is not always easy to assess the concept of "greatest good" or even "for the greatest number," so that one should proceed with the greatest deliberation to gather all the facts, also with the help of neutral or disinterested people who have some competence in this area, before going ahead. The same kind of advice ought to be followed by anyone else when faced with the decision of using the therapy in situations where the welfare of another is importantly involved.

These and other kinds of considerations that have come

to our attention, as a result of feedback and experiences we have had since the therapy first became public, have led us to understand better how much our interpersonal relationships play in both our significant problems, and in our imimplementation of Natural Therapy for them. And, since religion has some important considerations to contribute here, we are including our discussion of interpersonal relationships in this chapter.

RELIGION SHEDS LIGHT ON
INTERPERSONAL RELATIONSHIPS

In the early days of our research into human problems, we were quite convinced, like many therapists today, that guilt was at the basis of most personality problems, especially those that were associated with anxiety and inferiority. It is understandable, then, that, unlike those same therapists, we refused to accept the prevailing notion, introduced by psychiatrist Harry Stack Sullivan some time ago, that all problems were basically problems of interpersonal relationships. We had felt that guilt was basically the result of transgressing the Moral Law, and the widespread incidence of personal problems was indicative of that Law having been "written into *everyone's* heart."

As Natural Therapy developed it became clear to us, from a logical point of view, that, if the therapy had to do importantly with using ourselves primariy to help humankind, somehow the problem had to have something important to do with our relationship to others. And, on further contemplation of the matter, we were led to the idea that, if it was God or the Creator who placed this natural knowledge of His Law into everyone's consciousness, by that very act we were placed into an important relationship with that being or person called God. Thus, everyone was also inevitably, and at all times, somehow interacting with some other person, even if it was God Himself.

When, however, we were also led to the conclusion, which we have earlier described in this chapter when we discussed conscience, that the religious idea of an inborn knowledge of right and wrong is based principally for them on an incorrect translation of a Scripture passage, and is more adequately explained by Natural Therapy on the basis of differential inborn degree of conditionability, we had to reassess our previous acceptance of the idea that all problems have interpersonal relationship connotations, for we had apparently eliminated God as one of those persons. On further assessment, however, it finally became easy to substitute for God whatever person had ever sought to teach us some form or code of proper behavior, but only to the extent that such attempts were internalized by us, on the basis of how we were led to feel about them, as demonstrated earlier.

For Natural Therapy the idea that all problems have to do with interpersonal relationships poses no particular problem in assessing the cause of significant problems, but in their solution we are sometimes faced with decisions that present some difficulties. For these we have received some important assistance from religion, again, however, by using religious teachings somewhat differently than their proclaimers and adherents usually do.

It has come to our attention that, when former sufferers from significant problems have successfully used Natural Therapy to get control of their grandiosity and its attendant have-tos, they have not only realized what they now have to do with their natural selves, but they also now have the courage to try to do so, and are also quite anxious to do so. But very often they have to deal with some obstacles that stand in the way, among them the formidable one represented by the web of interpersonal relationships that were established earlier. We began to get questions like: "One doesn't just walk out on a spouse who opposes the new style of life, or does one?"

At first our advice, again based on our own religious background, was: "Of course not." To religious individuals anyway. But for some of them this was another formidable obstacle — their religion's view of such an action. All this was made worse when some of them, reflecting now upon why they married at all, why they married when they did, why they married the person they did marry, why they had children, why they even were religious, why they were church members, why they were active members, etc., noted that their acquired grandiosity had evidently played quite an important role. For some, then, all this presented some great dilemmas.

We had insisted earlier to our clients, especially the religious ones, that grandiosity wasn't all bad. We remember some of the responses we received to that. Most of them were to this effect: "If you really knew all the pain and suffering my grandiosity has caused me, you wouldn't say that." We can understand such reactions, knowing what a hell grandiosity can actually produce. At the same time, religious people do know that their religion teaches that even the seeming evil is sometimes used by God to bring about a greater good. Grandiosity especially makes that hard to accept. While, in our first book, we did already mention that grandiosity is sometimes a source of good, we have more to say about it in the next chapter of this one.

So, in retrospect, the assessment of what grandiosity had led them to, in the past, in the establishment of interpersonal ties, now only added to the trap in which many of those now found themselves who truly had learned who they were, and now wanted so very much to be who they were, in accordance with Natural Therapy. Since religion presented an additional obstacle for some, we searched for a solution there.

And we found a good one, and, as so often, it lay in a teaching of Jesus that is so often ignored by those who profess to be His followers. We know of no major religion that does not teach something, directly or by implication, quite similar.

Just about all of religion demands that their god be placed first in all of life. Biblical Christianity as well as Judaism make that their very first commandment, and their teachers also state that, if that commandment is kept, all the other ones will be kept also.

Thus any personal relationship that ever comes into conflict with allegiance to God and His will, must not only take second place, but may even have to be severed completely. In fact, Jesus once said that it would be necessary for those, who come to Him, to "hate" (loathe, despise) their father, mother, wife, children, brothers, and sisters, and even their own life. It's obvious, of course, that this strong reaction is to characterize the individual's attitude toward any relationships that interefere with discipleship to Jesus.

Now you already see how this might apply to the situation where any of those, with whom you have interpersonal relationships, oppose or try to prevent you from carrying out the Creator's prime purpose for your life. It is our advice, to you who find yourselves in this situation, to confront those individuals close to you with the reality of the situation for you. At the same time, it should not be difficult for the opposers to see their own great advantage in going along with you.

Actually, Jesus, who has been called a visionary for advocating what apparently are extreme measures, apparently impossible, turns out again to be a most astute psychologist, even as we pointed this out in a previous example. It is the theologians or the churches that have again turned this wonderful tool against their followers. The usual way that they implement this demand of Jesus is to apply it almost exclusively to allegiance to Christ as Savior. When they do apply it to living the moral life that He demands, they apply it to the letter of the Law instead of its spirit.

We cannot adequately explain this without discussing

the latter in a little further detail. Many people know that there is an ongoing controversy among religious people in this area.

It centers about concepts called moral relativity or situational ethics. Jesus cited at least one example of the need for situational considerations when He approved certain "violations" of the Sabbath. St. Paul nailed it down by saying that *agape* love was the essence of fulfilling the Law of God.

We hear a great deal about the word *agape,* a Greek term used quite extensively in the New Testament. Most Christians use it to mean "affection" especially of the undeserved variety. That has not made much sense to us, so in our research of religion, we tracked down the real meaning of that word, also through the fine help we received from the scholars at the University of California at Irvine who are involved with the Treasury of the Greek Language project there. This is perhaps the most valuable activity going on today especially for those interested in the study of the New Testament, for it is putting on tape every Greek word that was ever used in written documents, and the context in which it was used.

With their help also we were able to come up with this as the most fitting meaning for the word *agape,* when it is used to refer to interpersonal relationships: "an interest in someone with a view toward helping him." We are happy to state that others, who have been on a similar search for the word's meaning, and who are much more astute in Greek than we are, have come up with similar definitions.

Now see also how this fits so beautifully the Scripture declaration that *agape* love is the fulfilling of the Law. In other words, one cannot escape the fact that the real essence of fulfilling God's Law is not the putting into practice the exact prescribed action alone or even for the most part. That is often only what is known as legalism. It is rather performing, no matter in which precise manner, any action that will help the individuals involved, in the various areas that God's Law covers. It does not imply affection for those individuals, nor is it necessary to have affection for them. If one, in addition, does have affection (a different Greek word: *phile*), so much the better.

If you apply that meaning of *agape* toward others — God, your neighbor, your enemies — you will always be fulfilling God's Law. Even if you make a mistake in deciding what apparently is good for the other person. Criminal law in the United States recognizes this aspect of law fulfillment and violation. A crime is defined as a violation of the law, but *intent* has to be demonstrated.

Now we ought to be ready to place into proper perspective how this relates to our interpersonal relationships. We were discussing how ordinarily today religious leaders, while teaching that our first allegiance is to be toward our God and His will, often think in terms of fulfilling the letter of God's Law, which usually turns out to be observing the don'ts" of the commandments. When the "do's" of the commandments are mentioned, they again are mostly concerned with keeping the letter of the Law, but, even worse, they do not associate any of this with the command to put such obligations also ahead of our relationships with those who are our relatives or friends.

Now, obviously, practicing *agape,* and performing the "do's" of God's Law, is in essence nothing else but Natural Therapy, for it can only be done, and be done best, when we use our natural qualities, and all other abilities derived from them, primarily for the spiritual and temporal welfare of humankind. Thus again, if any of our interpersonal relationships interfere with our being able to do this to the best of our ability, then we are not only allowed, but are obligated to change them.

It is also important to note that those with whom we are closely associated can actually receive much more benefit for themselves if they allow us to use ourselves primarily as God has directed. For several reasons: they themselves no doubt will be important ones to whom our use of ourselves for others will be directed, and, second, they themselves may by our example be led to try to meet the prime purpose of *their* lives by learning to use themselves primarily to help others. This again goes to the heart of Natural Therapy, as we show so unmistakably later.

SACRED WRITINGS SUPPORT
NATURAL THERAPY

At this point we are citing a number of religious statements held in high regard by both religious and even some non-religious people, and which we feel remarkably support the principles of Natural Therapy. While they are almost exclusively from Biblical Christianity, they are rather characteristic of all major religions. In our study of religion over the years, which has included the chief teachings of the major religions, we have always been struck more by their similarity than their differences.

And this is what we should expect. Even the religions themselves tell us that we can learn much about God by observing nature and natural law in operation. So, while we set forth here some very relevant statements from the Scriptures, we are certain that adherents of non-Scripture based religions, and even those with no formal religious background at all, will find great agreement with them. In our projected book of readings in Natural Therapy we plan to include sacred writings of other major religions, as well as observations of astute observers of the religious scene. In our final section of this chapter we include a further relevant treatment of religion and natural law.

We did not intend, in this final version of our second book on our therapy, to include a treatment of the kinds of Bible passages that we list below, but at the special request of a rather significant number of religiously-oriented followers of Natural Therapy, who felt that they would be especially helpful to religious people, we have acceded to their request, if only in the limited way that we do so in what follows. The intention on our part is two-fold: to give

only a small sample of such relevant statements, and to indicate the added dimensions that we believe some important passages actually do have, in addition to what religion
has usually seen in them.

In our earlier book we gave some samples of what Scripture has to say about inborn conditionability, and,
although we have since then discovered even more important examples of the Biblical treatment of this basic component of the Natural Therapy system, we are not including them here. Instead we are concentrating here on
the other key component of the system, grandiosity, and
the Natural Therapy way of controlling it.

We have elsewhere mentioned the overwhelming number
of passages that speak of "pride" (really grandiosity) that
Scripture points out as the basis for all our big problems,
and there are a number of passages that importantly urge
humility. One can hardly read very far in the Scriptures
before coming across such passages, so we won't even
bother to cite any. But it might be of greater interest to indicate some passages that corroborate some of the special
uses to which our therapy has put them. All citations are
from the King James Version.

Take the statement that "whosoever exalteth himself
shall be abased," and put it into psychological terms, and
it turns out something like this: whoever is grandiose will
feel inferior — an unmistakable confirmation of our claim
that it is grandiosity that underlies our problems, for it is
that which produces the inferiority that is a prominent
symptom in many important problems.

Again, many feel that it is a lack of self-love that is at the
basis of so many important problems, and the word has
gotten around, aided by much of current therapy, that one
has to love one's self first, even before one can love
another. There is no such statement in Scripture, even as
there is no statement that any of our problems are due to
our poor self-image, our feelings of inferiority, our lack of
self-love, or even our feelings of guilt. While many reli-

gious people, and even their clergy, are still trying to use "Love thy neighbor as thyself" to prove otherwise, our more accurate and meaningful interpretation of that passage, given under our treatment of *agape* above, knocks out that erroneous use of that well-known passage.

The basic error is that they use the word *agape* to mean affection, which it does not, as we indicated earlier. There is another original Greek word for that — *phile.* But, as if it anticipated such an error, the Scripture has only one statement about self-love, in the sense of self-affection, when Paul warns Timothy that in the last days, "men shall be lovers of (have *phile* — affection — for) their own selves," and then adds a long list of extremely harmful behavior that will also be displayed by people. Acknowledging the Greek custom of putting the most important thing first in a sentence, one could very well state that all these kinds of destructive behaviors are being attributed to human self-affection, which is just another word for grandiosity.

We have already indicated elsewhere the New Testament's frequent and exclusive urging of the practice of *agape* (an interest in others with a view toward helping them) as the fulfilling of God's Law or will for human beings, and religious people have commonly taken this to mean that they should practice some kind of undeserved affection in their relationship to others. Ordinarily this kind of view of *agape* left them in the dark as to what specifically they ought to do, although they apparently know what it is telling them not to do.

Again it is largely the incorrect view of what *agape* really means that leaves them, not only in the dark, but somewhat befuddled. For example, if *agape* means, as commonly proclaimed, affection for the undeserving, then how does one apply that to God, to Whom above everyone else we are to show *agape?* God certainly is not undeserving, and He really doesn't need our affection anyway, even if we knew how to show it to Him.

But He does need our help if His unique plan to preserve the human race and to promote its progress is to be carried out. And He does not only need it, He orders it. This is really the thrust of His law, which Jesus summarized in the words:

> "Thou shalt love the Lord thy God with all thy heart, and with all thy soul, and with all thy mind.
> This is the first and great commandment. And the second is like unto it, Thou shalt love thy neighbor as thyself.
> On these two commandments hang all the law and the prophets."

Using the verb form of *agape* here correctly, this summary of the Law of God is literally saying that we must have an interest in God, above all, with a view toward helping Him, and in our fellowman, in the degree that we have it in ourselves, with a view toward helping him.

We, therefore, fulfill God's Law when we use ourselves, primarily, for the spiritual and temporal welfare of humankind. In both cases, in trying to do our duty to God and to our fellow humans, we end up doing the same thing. Jesus points this out when He also adds here: "The second (commandment) is like unto it (the first and greatest commandment)." And, of course, this is exactly what Natural Therapy says we must do to use our lives correctly.

Natural Therapy states that we must give of ourselves first for others, and this was commanded by Jesus long ago in the Sermon on the Mount, when He stated this general rule:

> "Give, and it shall be given unto you; good measure, pressed down, and shaken together, and running over, shall men give into your bosom."

But there are several other important things that this statement by Jesus points out that add considerably to our insights into our therapy. It promises that the giver will receive more for himself than what he gave to help others. This certainly is true from a Natural Therapy point of view, even if only such giving of one's self produces the control of one's significant problems, for which the therapy was originally designed.

But there is even more to be noted here, and that is that it is evident that even Jesus is holding out the promise of such great reward as a *motivation* to give first of ourselves. As Lord He simply could have said to His followers: "Give! because I want you to." He rather appeals to their self-interest in doing so, even as He and all of Scripture continually do. This certainly confirms our earlier concerns, that we had not made it clear enough in our first book, that our use of the therapy should not be attempted in an unselfish manner. Later on we implement this whole idea more fully and importantly.

There is even one more observation to make about this very meaningful passage. Jesus does not say that *God* would reward the giver; his fellow *humans* will. This is something also that we have mentioned in our earlier treatment of Natural Therapy, but now we see that we have not given this aspect the prominence it deserves. In our next and concluding section we show how this is also observable in natural law.

Before going on to that, we wish to add just this culminating exercise, which can serve both as a teaching device, as well as testing device, that relates to your understanding of Natural Therapy, as well as to the appreciation of what religion has contributed to its development, and what it can also contribute to a more successful implementation of it. Below are a few additional passages that we feel are highly significant to the therapy. Take a few moments to try to determine why we feel that way about them:

> "Whosoever will be great among you,
> let him be your minister: and

whosoever will be chief among you,
let him be your servant.''

"Blessed are the merciful:
for they shall obtain mercy.''

"Train up a child *in the way he
should go* (literally: *according
to his nature*): and when he is
old, he will not depart from it.''

"Perfect *love (agape)* casteth
out fear.''

"*Charity (agape)* vaunteth not itself, is not puffed up.''

"And *now* (can mean: *for this life*)
abideth faith, hope, and charity *(agape),*
these three; but the greatest of
these is *charity (agape).*''

"He that humbleth himself shall be
exalted.''

"Whosoever will save his life
shall lose it; and whosoever will
lose his life *for my sake* (literally: *for Me*) shall find it.''

"If any be a hearer of the word,
and not a doer, he is like unto
a man beholding his natural face
in a glass, and straightway for-
getteth what manner of man he was.''

"He hath showed thee, O man,
what is good;
and what doth the Lord require of thee,
but to do justly,
and to love mercy,
and to walk humbly with thy God?''

"As every man hath received *the* (lit-

erally: *a) gift* (has to be: *natural
gift*), even so minister the same
one to another."

RELIGION CONFIRMS NATURAL LAW

We have invoked two concepts — conscience and
natural law — as important in Natural Therapy, and in this
section we seek to clarify how and why this is so. It is our
contention that religion confirms natural law, as we have
already implied when we said earlier that, for many,
natural law is just another name for God.

There is very good evidence that there is a natural law
operating in the universe, in the minds of some a law that
originated through evolution or was created and is enforced by a Creator, a law that, in general, operates on the
principle that you reap what you sow, you get what you
deserve, and you can take what you want but you have to
pay for it.

It is most evident in its negative aspects, for negative-
type phenomena have a more powerful impact upon
humans than positive ones. A Hitler ignores the sanctity of
human life and is destroyed ignominiously in the process.
You lose your temper, kick the door, and you injure your
ankle or leg in the process. You envy or hate, and you
develop tension and physical and emotional problems in
abundance. You fail to brush your teeth, or in some other
way to take care of your physical body, and your health
suffers as a result. You commit a crime, and you fear getting caught.

Despite all this, there are those that, because of their
grandiosity, are led to feel that they can do anything they
want and get away with it. The result is that they have
problems of all kinds. Not only does the *individual* have to
pay the price of his grandiosity-induced actions, *society*
pays, too.

This natural law also has its positive aspects. This part of
the law states that, if you work hard, and even make sacri-

fices, you will be rewarded, to that extent at least. The student who studies hard is likely to receive good grades and has a better chance for a good job after graduation than the one who doesn't. The person who takes care of his health is likely to avoid much illness. The individual who performs his job well and faithfully is likely to be promoted. But there are individuals, who, because of their grandiosity, are led to think that they can do otherwise and still get ahead. The result is problems.

There is also one specific part of that general law that states that, if you give priority to the welfare of others, you yourself will be rewarded, again to the extent that you do so, and often beyond that. An Albert Schweitzer gives of himself primarily to the physical welfare of the deprived natives in a relatively-unknown small spot on the globe in far-off Africa, and he is hailed as one of the greatest persons that ever lived. An employee works primarily in the interest of his employer, and he becomes an officer of the company. A teacher, who gives herself primarily to the welfare of her students, is highly respected by them, receives their cooperation, and is also held in honor by the community. But there are those, who, because of their grandiosity, think they can get such rewards without such service and get away with it. The result is problems.

We stated at the outset of this section that natural law generally supports Natural Therapy. It does so in two major ways. It illustrates, without a doubt, that an unwillingness to do what is necessary to do to avoid problems (and this is nothing else but a manifestation of grandiosity) produces problems, and that using one's self primarily to help others avoids them, or solves them if they occur. How it does this is generally quite obvious, even for example, in the case of the individual who loses his temper, kicks the door, and injures his ankle. If he were not grandiose, he would not ordinarily become frustrated to that extent.

But, someone says, natural law does not always work the way it is expected to. Sometimes those we help repay us with trouble. Crime does seem to pay at times. Some leaders in athletics claim that nice guys finish last. Some who ignore the welfare of others often seem to prosper, while one who gives priority to the welfare of others often seems to go unrewarded; in fact, he sometimes appears to have an even greater share of hardships than others.

When one can observe only the surface manifestations of such atypical results, it may appear that natural law is not that dependable. We contend, however, that if one could discover what goes on beneath the surface, or if one can see the phenomena in long-term perspective, one could be convinced that natural law always works.

The very fact that our universe, and specifically humankind, continues to survive and prosper is mute evidence that natural law does work, and works so well that enough individuals can discern it, and thus be led to act accordingly, part of which involves the use of themselves to bring about such great results.

There is another consideration here that needs to be pointed out. It is also grandiosity that leads some humans to try to discredit natural law, as it pertains to human behavior, because it has led them to dictate what results we ought to have when we try to observe it, never realizing that a Higher Intelligence operates the law and knows better what the specific form these outcomes should take for the benefit of the individuals involved. Again, the solution is Natural Therapy to control that grandiosity.

Religion, of course, adds to the validity of natural law by contending that it is not just some rather impersonal and not-altogether-reliable rule of unclear or mysterious origin. It is looked upon as a precise, definite, and wholly reliable law that was instituted and is enforced by a loving Creator. So we should not be surprised that Scripture and the teachings of the major religions also hold us responsible for our actions, and openly promise or threaten that we will reap what we sow. Thus the heart of Natural Therapy, which holds that we must first sow, if we are to reap solutions to our earthly problems, is reinforced again.

In addition, before we knew the divine nature of natural law, we could not adequately account for the seeming exceptions to that law in the ways that we have attempted to. Now we know also that seeming exceptions are no exceptions at all, but are only the better outcomes for us as a result of the superior intelligence and judgment behind them. It would be only grandiosity on our part that prevents us from enjoying the benefits of that knowledge.

It is also and only grandiosity that prevents some religious people from seeing and admitting that even religious people are subject to their God's natural law, and thus they are led to use religion as magic for their problems, in the ways we have described and deplored earlier. If such would take time to observe natural law in operation all around them, they would see that the sun shines on the evil and on the good, and that it rains both upon the just and the unjust, as the Scriptures so plainly state it.

Thus one might say that, for the non-religious person, natural law confirms the existence of some superior Omnipotence or Omniscience at work in the universe, and, for the religious individual, religion confirms the existence of natural law. And in that no one loses, and everyone gains, for in either or both instances, whoever is involved receives greater motivation, and even inspiration, to be the person he was intended to be, and is led further down the path to his life's fulfillment.

We've now come to the end of our brief treatment of what we have learned about our therapy since we first brought it to the attention of others. In all that follows, we describe the updated therapy to which all this has thus far brought us.

chapter **5**

The Real Problem —
Have-Tos

WE ISOLATE THE HAVE-TO

In an earlier chapter we described how we were led to the discovery of have-tos principally through the feedback we received from some of those who thought about trying the therapy, or who actually gave it a good try. Either they plainly told us that the therapy was "too hard," or we discovered that some, who used it with considerable initial success, found themselves trying to take a short cut to gain ongoing success.

Our first analysis of this phenomenon had led us to conclude that we had not emphasized the fact that the therapy was designed primarily for the purpose of helping individuals overcome their significant problems. It seemed that those who were having a hard time implementing it, and continuing with it, had the impression that they needed to go about it with absolutely no self-interest at all, and it's certainly understandable that grandiose people especially could find little motivation to try it, or to go on with it, unless they had immediate and dazzling results, a highly unlikely outcome.

We tried to counter that impression, not by promising those kinds of results, but emphasizing that, while they had to give first and very much of themselves, they would receive more in return for themselves, even if it were only the ability to control their significant problems. And that therefore they should not at all try to go about the therapy unselfishly. One way that we suggested, that might help them to get the correct feeling about what they were to do, was to have them concentrate, not on the individuals being helped by their activity, but on the help itself. We urged them to be concerned mostly about maximizing themselves and in any other way to maximize the help itself that they were rendering.

When they attacked their task in that way, there was an improvement in their attitude toward it, but it did not seem to be the final answer. And as we analyzed that further, we concluded that the improvement was due mainly to the fact that we had satisfied one of their have-tos, the have-to that things should be easy for them. So we should not have been surprised that our little strategem of turning the focus away from other people to the maximizing of *ourselves* and the contribution *we* were making, was only helping by indulging a have-to.

In effect, therefore, we were only doing what so many therapists do today, which make many of their clients feel that they are being helped, when they tell them to assert themselves, build up their own self-esteem, think of their interests first, think positively (which usually means — think of those things that you desire for yourself), etc. Everyone feels better when he is stroked, but, in everyday life, hardly anyone enjoys the luxury of eternal stroking by others, and, sooner or later, those, who think that stroking one's self and stroking others is most important, have to take time out for other important activities demanded for survival, if only to stroke somebody else, or to find others who will carry on the stroking that others give them, when those others leave to find more stroking for themselves. When health authorities tell us that strokes are on the increase and becoming a bigger health problem, the same could be said of the kind of strokes we're discussing here. We shudder everytime we see that common bumper sticker: "Have you hugged your kid today?" We think that it ought to say: "Unless your kid is still a mere infant, have you taught your kid to get along without your hug today?" Because, when they get out on their own later, they're going to find more muggers than huggers out there.

Anyway, as a result of our attempts to determine how we could help our clients overcome the feeling that the therapy was too difficult, we were gaining considerable respect for the have-to phenomenon. While up till then we looked upon have-tos as important ingredients in grandiosity, we now began to think of them as important in their own right. And it wasn't long before we began to see the true relationships and progression involved. This we describe in the following section.

Before going on to that, we would like to mention a newspaper article (*Los Angeles Times,* October 1, 1979) that made us wonder why it took so long for us to see this. Here a daughter of the well-known entertainer Carol Burnett gives her diagnosis of why she had become a drug addict: "I'm *compulsive* and I'm extremist, and I did have *a big ego* (italics ours)." You'll see from what follows why we think she has it right.

NOT-TOOS, WANT-TOS, AND HAVE-TOS

As a result of our further study of the have-to phenomenon, we have come up with the following scheme, which depicts quite clearly the three major categories of human beings, when classified according to their basic attitudes toward their particular life situation:

1. Individuals who generally accept the way things are for them.

2. Individuals who desire to have things to be better for them.

3. Individuals who insist that everything has to be the best for them.

Of course, it is understood that their own assessment of their situation is based upon how they personally feel about it.

Those of our readers who have been reading with understanding can easily describe these three types in Natural Therapy terms, and would do so in the following manner:

1. Moderately conditionable (ambiverted) individuals who are naturally moderately-emotional.

2. Easily-conditionable or difficult-to-condition individuals who are naturally highly emotional, but who have not developed grandiosity (non-grandiose introverts and extraverts).

3. Same as 2 above, but grandiose.

It is, of course, also understood that the degree, to which that characteristic exists in each of these three groupings, correlates with the degree, of the types of conditionability common to that grouping, that any particular individual in the grouping possesses it.

More succinctly, these three types might be characterized by the following expressed feelings regarding changes for the better in their life situations:

1. I'm *not too* interested. (Short for: I might be ininterested if it's not too much trouble for me.)

2. I *want to*. (Short for: I feel very much that I'd like to have them.)

3. I *have to*. (Short for: I'll accept and settle for nothing less.)

We've all seen these kinds of attitudes commonly as

typical of the kinds of reactions that humans display regarding various life's situations with which they are confronted, and each of them has in it the possibility for the development of some problem for the individual confronted. Of course, the severity of the problem would differ for each of them, even though they all might take the same kind of action in that situation.

Suppose that each of them had an opportunity to make an investment in a project that is almost certain to make them a considerable profit. None of them has the money to make such an investment, but all of them have good enough credit ratings that might induce some lender to loan them money. The *not-too* doesn't even try to borrow the money, after learning that he has to come to the lender with practically all his financial history, and he doesn't really feel ambitious enough to go through all that, nor does he have the desire to skip the TV football game to investigate the investment further.

The *want-to* is very much interested, does his homework on the investment possibility, and even gathers up all the information the lender desires. The lender, however, turns him down, feeling that he would need more security for the loan. And Mr. Want-To is disappointed, but feels that he doesn't want it that badly that he should put more time and effort into it, and then possibly receive only more disappointment. He makes a few phone calls only to several other possible lenders to determine their general attitudes, but, when they also are not evidently good prospects for a loan, he forgets the whole idea.

The *have-to* individual combs the woods for a prospective lender, comes, armed to the teeth with his whole financial record and testimonials to his integrity, to a number of prospective lending agencies, and even browbeats his wife into consenting to a possible third mortgage on the house (they're still paying on the second mortgage, taken out for a similar sure-thing investment that never did pay off). Turned down time and again, he finally gives up only after all sources of help have been explored, pressured, begged, etc. without result.

All three were originally interested in improving their financial situation, but all three took different steps to pursue it. The outcomes for all of them were the same — no one could seize the opportunity that the investment evidently held out for them. But there were great differences in how all this affected each of them.

Certainly everyone knows the degree of tension that characterizes the way each of them went about to do something about the opportunity. And we all have seen too often both the degree of emotional upset, and the length of time that it has to be endured, as a result of the way each of them felt about the goal to which their different activity was directed. In sum, the entire incident culminated in a significant problem for only one of them, Mr. Have-To. And we wouldn't be surprised if the sorry memory of it did not continue to color all his remaining days, unless, of course, he learned to control his have-tos.

The kinds of differentiations we have included here, together with our earlier description of have-tos in a previous chapter, should leave no doubt in your mind about our definition of the term have-to. Nor should you need any additional evidence to indicate that they can really produce the significant problems that we claim they do. In the remaining sections of this chapter we dwell on their development for the purpose, here, of mainly preparing you for dealing successfully with them, and for the future, of helping to avoid their development at all.

HOW HAVE-TOS DEVELOP

It should be quite evident that the two key components of the Natural Therapy system — inborn degree of conditionability by external influences, and grandiosity — are the necessary ingredients in the development of have-tos. In our first presentation of the therapy it would appear that the development of significant problems followed this basic scheme:

> extremes of conditionability + early socialization + grandiosity + crisis situation = significant problems.

From what we have learned and added since, the following now presents a more complete and more accurate scheme:

> extremes of conditionability + high emotionality + early socialization + grandiosity + have-tos + crisis situation = significant problems

Readers will recognize the alterations of the original presentation of the therapy in the following: the greater importance of the inborn high emotionality of those at the extremes of conditionability (easy and difficult types), the addition of the have-tos, and the suggestion that grandiosity itself may not be a significant problem (note that we say *may*).

It is clear that the inborn high emotionality, so necessary if those that have it are to carry out the leadership tasks for which they were originally designed, is not a have-to. It is more a kind of want-to. But this inborn high emotionality, with the addition of the development of grandiosity, is what makes the emotionality a have-to, or changes the want-to into a have-to. So there is no have-to without grandiosity. But the following also now needs to be considered.

GRANDIOSITY NOT NECESSARILY A SIGNIFICANT PROBLEM?

In our original presentation of our therapy one could get the impression that grandiosity and the significant problems it produced were almost one and the same, the problems being the form in which grandiosity expressed itself.

As stated before, we have since declared that grandiosity may not be all bad, and we have sought to explain that further in this book. And now that idea fits neatly into what we are saying here. But one important correction needs to be made: we must use the term have-to instead of grandiosity, for it is the have-tos that really cause significant problems.

Actually, in our early presentation of the therapy, we did indicate quite clearly that only in a situation of crisis of some kind could the grandiosity produce significant problems. This, of course, accounts for the time differential that is clearly seen in the appearance of significant problems, even though, in just about every case, grandiosity develops in individuals in the early years of life.

But that consideration, in addition to the fact that it is finally the have-tos that produce such problems, does not mean that the grandiose individual will not have a problem. He does have problems, more problems than non-grandiose individuals, but they need not be significant ones, at least for the individual involved. Such problems may be labeled as significant by others, however.

Here's a typical example. A grandiose easily-conditioned child is enrolled in kindergarten, and there he usually sits quietly, usually by himself, does not socialize with the others, does a lot of daydreaming, and doesn't seem to be happy. At first he would rather stay home, but after he attends a few weeks, gets better acquainted with the teacher and the other pupils and the routine, he doesn't object to going, and, when questioned by his mother, he says that he likes it.

Meantime, while he may loosen up in his former unassertive ways, he continues to be rather quiet and does not participate very freely, or to any great extent, on his own. The mother is quite upset when the boy brings home the first report of his performance, or, when she visits on parent-teacher day, she is informed that the teacher is worried about his asocial and timid performance. More often than not, the mother basing her conclusions on her own observation of the child in his interactions with siblings and next-door playmates, feels that the teacher is mistaken, or even just brainwashed by all this modern child-psychology. And, to be sure, the child never develops any important educational problems, or maybe any other significant problems, all the rest of his life.

That last part is highly unlikely, for there is hardly even a statistical probability that any human can avoid a crisis situation if he lives a normal length of life. But, until that crisis moment arrives, he may very well have not become a victim of a serious problem. We remember very well how so many were very much alarmed at the high rate of breakdowns that occurred in our armed forces during World War II, especially when it was evident that most of them broke down already in the States, and not as much overseas and in combat. As a chaplain, we were often in the decision-making chain, whose reponsibility was to designate those who might have to be discharged for those reasons.

The crisis situation brought on by the war often served to hasten the onset of significant problems for those grandiose individuals destined to develop such problems sooner or later in their lifetime. It is for this reason that it pains us to see some individuals dismiss what we try to tell them about grandiosity simply because they have never had a significant problem. How often we have heard these same kinds of individuals, whom we counsel, say: "If only I can get back to what I used to be!" But the truth more likely is that now they are finally learning who they really always were, but never knew it. And that gives us the more pleasant moments, when we can show them how to capitalize on who they really are, instead of short-circuiting themselves as they have been doing.

We have gone into some detail to demonstrate that grandiosity is "not all that bad" more or less to modify the impression that we gave, up until more recently, that it was grandiosity that was the real culprit. Now we want to go further to repeat that it is finally the have-tos that produce significant problems, so that all that we have said in this section about grandiosity applies to have-tos. While have-tos do not develop without grandiosity, it is not only grandiosity that produces the have-tos. Further, where there is grandiosity there are also have-tos, for have-tos cannot exist without grandiosity. This becomes more clear in the following concluding section of this chapter.

HAVE-TOS ARE THE REAL PROBLEM

In our first presentation of Natural Therapy we did not make clear the relationship between the high emotionality of those at the extremes of conditionability and the grandiosity which they were predisposed to develop. We had left open the possibility that it was the grandiosity that produced the high emotionality. In this book, we not only recognize their independence, but also their coming together to form the have-tos that finally produce significant problems.

The high emotionality, where it exists in those that are not grandiose, produces the want-tos that enable them to carry out their leadership tasks, for which they were designed, with just the right amount of concern. Any more than that, produced by grandiosity, might easily distort for them the realities inherent in their carrying out their leadership tasks correctly, and bring on more significant problems than those for which their leadership was needed.

Thus again, it is the have-tos, the compulsions to act in accordance with what our grandiosity has indicated to us is best for us, that are the real problem. And the remaining chapters are designed to point out how Natural Therapy deals with them to solve the real problem.

chapter **6**

Resolution of the Have-To Problem:
You Really Don't Have To!

RECOGNIZE THE ESSENCE OF THE
HAVE-TO PROBLEM

If you have wondered why we used so much space in this book to try to describe what have-tos are and how they develop, you can understand the reason when you read this chapter, which is really the heart of this book. After all, when significant problems have gone unsolved for so long because we really have evidently failed to discover the underlying cause, and when we have good evidence to indicate that we have finally come upon it, we would be downright irrational if we did not try to describe that cause and its cure as clearly and completely as possible. For the final evidence lies in implementing that information to resolve important problems, and, in a primarily self-help book of this kind, any failure to describe or understand that information will surely result in an equivalent failure in achieving success in such an important endeavor.

We've already described the essence of have-tos. Here we try to describe the essence of the have-to *problem*.

What must one do to modify, control, or even eliminate have-tos? We really don't know until we can define the essence of the problem.

We have gone to some length to indicate that have-tos are the product of inborn high emotionality plus grandiosity. Now you can understand more fully why we have been so insistent on the necessity for accepting a biological basis for the production of degree of conditionability, and for what have been demonstrated to be, especially by Eysenck and his associates, concomitants of such conditionability, in this case high emotionality. If it is biologically-derived, it cannot basically be changed.

Incidentally, the prescription and administration of drugs to modify high emotionality, which occurs so commonly in the treatment of significant problems by medical professionals, is certainly a very high testimonial to the common involvement of high emotionality in significant problems. While such practices may be helpful and even necessary at times in the earlier phases of treatment, they tend to obscure the underlying cause of the problems. Tranquilizers and other mood-altering drugs are usually administered in the belief that it is the *problem* that is caus-- ing the high emotionality that is so highly visible in such situations. And, of course, when such high emotionality is modified and controlled to some extent by such medication, no further thought is given to what part the high emotionality might play even in the etiology of the problem.

Thus we have this common but deplorable situation, which so many of us are trying to change these days, in which such drugs, with their tranquilizing and often-stupifying effects, prevent those afflicted with some serious functional problem from mustering up enough will and energy to go into action to do those things, like using Natural Therapy, by which alone they can ever expect to control their problems.

You can understand, then, that to know, that inborn high emotionality cannot be changed, enables one to avoid that big trap that has been inadvertently set by modern therapy approaches. Much of our counseling so often has to be devoted, at the very outset, to extricating victims that have been so entrapped, and it is both difficult and time-consuming.

In addition, evolution or a Creator implanted high emotionality in certain individuals, not for the purpose of creating problems or aggravating them, but to help solve them. It is always a great joy for us in our counseling, when, after our clients have acquired enough control of their problem to decrease their use of tranquilizing medication, we see them attacking the remaining areas of their problem with the enthusiasm that only high emotionality can provide.

Eliminating inborn high emotionality from the essence of the have-to problem, we are left only with the other component that produces have-tos — grandiosity. So, we were right in our very first presentation of our therapy, when we aimed it at grandiosity. While have-tos are the real problem, they can only be satisfactorily dealt with by controlling the only controllable component involved in its production — grandiosity. And, if you still don't know for sure what we mean by grandiosity, before going on, take time to turn back to chapter one and review what we have to say about it there.

DON'T TRY TO ELIMINATE SELF-INTEREST

Remember that in this chapter we are dealing only with the have-to problem, and we have just stated that, to finally deal with that, we must do something about grandiosity. It would be great if we could plunge right into that, as we did in our early presentation of Natural Therapy, but we soon find that this is not easy to do. We first have to get around our have-tos enough to be willing to tackle grandiosity. That is why this is the most important chapter in this book. If we can't get past our have-to barriers, the therapy won't even be attempted, at least seriously enough to be effective.

There's no doubt in our minds, a result of our experiences with those who attempt to use Natural Therapy, that it's quite difficult to separate the therapy — using one's natural self primarily to help others — from the ideal, generally held by all of humankind, of unselfish behavior. While we have noted, among those who are acquainted with Natural Therapy, a ready acquiescence with the altruistic principle involved, it seems that few really wanted to live according to it.

We have speculated about this phenomenon and have come upon a few explanations for it. A few years back we would have attributed the negative reaction to what was viewed positively as a good to two common theological tenets. In the doctrine of the natural knowledge of right and wrong, one knew intuitively that altruistic behavior was right. And from the doctrine of original sin, one would also be inclined to rebel against indulging in such behavior.

With our definitive view of the natural knowledge of right and wrong discussed in chapter four, we could not attribute the favorable feeling toward altruistic behavior to that. And, with our amplified view of original sin, which we explain in the following chapter, we could not go along with that as an explanation for the unwillingness to practice altruism.

Perhaps it has been our own more frequent interacting with the non-religious world in recent years that has led us to see that a large segment of the population does not apparently believe in the desirability of altruistic behavior. That, in brief, would indicate that some, because of their kind of conditionability, do not internalize any conditioning in that direction.

What about the phenomenon, widely visible, in which altruistic behavior is applauded and given high acclaim? Someone may answer that altruistic behavior happens so seldom that it's news. That may explain why it is highly publicized, but it doesn't explain why it is often highly praised. A Freudian-type explanation might suggest that it is a way of society atoning for its guilt for its failure to practice such behavior. With our view of guilt feelings, given elsewhere, the continual and ongoing indulgence in such high acclaim for altruistic behavior suggests to us that it is rather a reaction engendered by grandiosity on the part of those who do the acclaiming.

What we are suggesting is that the high regard for altruistic behavior for its own sake, in effect raising it to the status of natural law, is hardly tenable. In fact, those who have tried to examine it objectively, have usually ended up by concluding that such behavior is essentially completely selfish. In that sense it would harmonize with natural law.

By virtue of our survival, every one of us has undeniable evidence of our own basic self-interest. Thus, for survival, which is the intention of both evolution and creation, one can hardly indulge in any behavior that does not have in it a greater or lesser amount of self-interest. One can even discern it in instances where one individual gives up his life to save another. Our very survival, humanly speaking, is dependent upon our self-interest.

Such an idea is hard for a religious person to accept, and yet every religion is based upon that self-interest. While Christians are at first shocked when they are told that their faith in Christ for forgiveness and eternal life is basically selfish, they can never come up with any evidence that it is not. And we have already indicated, in chapter four, how so often and unmistakably the sacred writings appeal to the reward found in obeying God's commands, an obvious inducement to do so.

And now along comes Natural Therapy to emphasize that it is God's or evolution's stated or obvious plan to give to humans the highest earthly reward — the avoidance of significant earthly problems, as well as the great satisfaction and the high self-esteem that comes from fulfilling the highest purpose of one's human life — for using themselves primarily in the interest of the welfare of all humankind. In Natural Therapy the one who practices it is by far the greatest beneficiary of it.

In view of such considerations, everyone should approach his decision about possibly participating in the therapy with the full realization that, while he is asked to use himself primarily to help others, he is in reality helping himself above all others. And, if anyone decides to participate, he should continually remind himself that, the more fully he participates, the more he is helping himself. Behind every have-to is the belief that one's present behavior is the best way to get one's needs fulfilled. In what we have just stated in this section we are saying that this simply is not true. To put it another way, if you feel that you just have to act as you do for your own self-interest, even though it is producing some big problems for you, then we are saying: *You really don't have to!*, for there is a better way to act in your own interest.

STOP BEING DEPENDENT UPON OTHERS

If you examine your have-tos closely, you will make the surprising discovery that they are, to a large extent, the result of your dependence upon others. We had already forewarned you about this when we stated earlier that all problems are problems of interpersonal relationships.

Now, we are not saying that humans can do without any relationships to others. John Donne had it right when he stated that no one is an island. Neither are we saying that we should not depend on anyone else for anything. Donne had it right here, too, when he also said that, when bells tolled for anyone, they were tolling for everyone, for all of us evidently lose something when someone dies. Certainly that is especially true in the light of an underlying principle of Natural Therapy, the one that holds that the principal purpose of our earthly life is to use ourselves primarily for the welfare of all humankind; all of us therefore are included, on both the giving and the receiving end.

But in this matter of our dependency upon others, we are referring to our dependence upon others as sources and determiners of our feelings about ourselves, our self-image. If you examine your have-tos, you will find that many of the things, if not all of them, they compel you to do, are designed, directly or indirectly, somehow to get someone else to act in ways that you feel they need to act, if your needs and interests are to be met as you want them met.

Significant problems between husband and wife, parents and children, brothers and sisters, employer and employee, pastor and parishioner, teacher and pupil, etc., are all the result of one, or another, or even all, in any dependency relationship, feeling that they have to act or react, the way they do in it, for their own best interest, all of which is finally designed for the maintenance or enhancement of the self-image of each of those performing in the have-to manner.

It should be self-evident, except perhaps to the grandiose, that such dependency for such purposes is an exceedingly precarious arrangement, for, sooner or later, those on whom we depend often let us down, and most often in those very areas for which we primarily, though often unconsciously, establish and maintain those dependent relationships. While many of those interdependent relationships are so much easier to get into than out of, such as those that have come about through marriage, parenthood, and the like, and one might feel it necessary to maintain them for the greater good of the most individuals involved, we can certainly stop depending upon any other individual, organization, institution, or whatever, as a source of our image of ourselves.

Whether we sever any relationships in the process or not, we can certainly cease depending upon anyone or anything in them for our feelings about ourselves. To acquire and maintain an independent self-image we should learn to depend only on what *we* do, and not what anyone else does.

We need to become independent of anyone or anything else for our self-image.

It is not unusual, when we counsel a religious person with a very difficult problem, that the client will say: "I guess only God can cure me." Our usual reply is: "The chances of that happening are highly improbable, at least in the way that you are evidently envisioning it, which involves the performance of a miracle." Humanly speaking again, to get on top of your significant problem, it will have to be you that finally does it.

So, here again, while your problem-producing behavior has originated with your feeling that you *have to* have another person think, say, or do certain things that will maintain or enhance your own self-image, the evidence we have presented to you here is really saying to you: *You really don't have to!*

YOU ARE NOW READY FOR UPDATED NATURAL THERAPY

We know of no other effective way of solving the have-to problem than the ways we have suggested in this brief chapter. There's no doubt that, on the basis of all that we have said about have-tos in this book, the future will yield many more additional ways of dealing with the problem. The very fact, that humans have not been able to deal very successfully with significant problems in the past, can very well explain the lack of information about have-tos at the present time, and account even more for the even greater lack of information of how to deal successfully with the problem.

If you still feel that you are not as ready as you'd like to be to tackle the full Natural Therapy program that can culminate in the control or even elimination of your big problems, then carefully reread this chapter. It's short. It won't take you long. And it has all the ingredients to hit you hard at the very point where you now really are.

Because of your big problems, your grandiosity is showing loud and clear. If you haven't seen it before, you now can no longer hide it from yourself, for we have exposed its presence in your have-tos.

Okay, you're so interested in yourself. We address ourselves to that in the best possible ways in this chapter. We first go along with your great self-interest by telling you that you are right in having your greatest interest in your own welfare. So we've removed any guilt you might have had for that amid all this talk about the greater importance of something called altruism. Self-interest is even an important motivating factor for the best of religion. It's no longer a have-to for you; it's rather a natural and even a spiritual expectation for human behavior.

Let's go on. Your grandiosity constantly tells you that you are really a great person, better than most. But why are you always trying to manipulate people to make them see your greatness, too? Or, are you really not that sure that you are as great as you think you are? So we're challenging you here, mostly to prove to yourself where the truth lies about your greatness. If you really are so great, then quit trying to use others in the ways you have. In other words, prove that *you really don't have to!*

If you are really interested in your own welfare, and if you accept our challenge to stand on your own two feet, then plunge into the program outlined in the next chapter, knowing that, if and when you do, you'll find your have-tos changing into want-tos.

chapter **7**

Natural-Therapy Updated:
Changing Have-Tos
To Want-Tos

HERE WE PUT IT ALL TOGETHER

This chapter is designed to put all that we have said in this book into a form that presents to the reader an effective treatment for all significant problems. It is a step-by-step presentation that includes also a brief description of what the user of our updated therapy may expect when he or she takes the various steps suggested. We do not mean to imply that everyone using Natural Therapy will always have precisely the same results when taking a particular step. We mention merely the minimal result a user should obtain before going on to the next step.

In this way we also hope to impress the reader with the importance of following as precisely as possible each step in the therapy. There are no short-cuts in obtaining results. Remember, grandiose individuals always want to take short-cuts. Take our word for it — what we present here is the *shortest*-cut for your kind of problem.

NECESSARY PRELIMINARIES

On the basis of our previous experiences with those attempting to use Natural Therapy we have discovered that it is all-important, from the very beginning, to meet six important prerequisites, without which the prospective user will not be able to approach the task with any reasonable chance for success. As we list these six prerequisites in this section the reader cannot fail to realize their great importance. In fact, when one fulfills these prerequisites, one is already halfway to the control of one's significant problem, for, as the old saying has it, what's well begun is half done.

We begin, then, with the *first prerequisite,* which is that one must accept, without any significant reservations, at least these three components of the Natural Therapy system — biological determinism (specifically and especially inborn degree of conditionability by influences from without), grandiosity (specifically and especially its have-to or compulsive aspects), and the necessity to maximize and use natural qualities (especially degree of conditionability) for one's self primarily by assisting others to similarly maximize and use their natural selves.

The *second prerequisite* is that one must believe as fully as possible that the therapy will accomplish what it is designed to do for the control or even elimination of any significant problem to which it is properly applied. Because there are so many approaches to problems today that are quite unusual and even bizarre, this prerequisite needs a great deal of further elaboration. It is not made to imply any kind of mystical idea that there is some mysterious force at work, that will not go into action unless one has implicit faith that such a force is at work in it. Rather it is an attempt to face the easily-demonstrated truth that, what one perceives as real, is real in its consequences. Or, as we usually tell our students, perception is reality. In this instance we are implying that, the more faith we have in the therapy, the more zealously we will practice it, the more rapidly we will achieve results, the results we achieve will be better, and the more easily we will be able to see them.

Those that we have counseled are aware of our insistence on that kind of confidence in the therapy, for some of them we have refused to counsel until they could achieve a measure of such confidence. Often the situation of the client is so painful that he or she is quite ready and eager to accept the therapy without question, and, not surprisingly, some of these have achieved excellent results so early that it has been difficult for us at times not to expect also an early setback, which seldom really ever occurred.

We have also known some who wanted very much to believe, but, for various reasons, frequently because they had tried so many other therapy approaches without success, they found it difficult to do so. To such we have often said: "Try it, and you will see." But that's not the best way to achieve the necessary faith, for any trial without adequate faith in it, is bound to be rather half-hearted and thus achieve also less-than-satisfactory outcomes.

Now, more often than not, we have advised the doubters to act as if the therapy were completely true, and the results have often been phenomenal. There is no mystery about this kind of approach, and religion uses it all the time. It's just another demonstration of the fact that perception is reality. We're saying: "Deliberately make believe that it is true, and you will find it easy to implement it in an adequate manner." When this is done, some early favorable results are achieved, enough to turn the make-believe into reality.

The *third prerequisite* is that one must be fully conscious of and be firmly convinced of the fact that no one else but one's self will be the one who has to implement the therapy completely. We have indicated earlier that, for earthly problems, the statistical probability of any miracle happening is so remote that, to expect anything like that to occur can only lead to a less-than-adequate implementation of the therapy. The sooner one learns, in the kinds of problems for which the therapy is designed, that "if it is to be, it is up to me," as someone has so nicely stated it, the sooner one is ready to tackle the therapy properly. By this time the reader fully understands the implications of this important prerequisite for the ones that become enmeshed in significant problems — the grandiose.

The *fourth important prerequisite* might very well be the most important of all — one must fully understand at least the three essential components of the therapy we listed already in the first prerequisite. The lack of such understanding may very well account for the failure to meet the three previous requirements. We place this fourth prerequisite here mainly to imply that this is something that one needs to be aware of throughout the implementation of the therapy. When one does not seem to be experiencing that the therapy is working the results it has promised at any particular stage or in any particular area of the therapy, then more often than not this is due to some failure in understanding it adequately.

Full understanding thus is necessary to fulfill the three previous requisites listed above, and then for effectively implementing it. No one should begin the therapy proper without feeling a good deal of confidence that he or she rather fully understands at least these essentials: inborn conditionability, grandiosity and its have-tos, and using one's natural self properly. Such confidence may come only after careful reading and rereading of this book, perhaps also enlisting the help of others for fuller understanding of it.

A *fifth prerequisite* is the necessity to accept the fact that it is grandiosity, and nothing but grandiosity, that has caused the significant problem that one is experiencing. We take for granted that the one contemplating using the therapy has been able to isolate any physical cause that may be wholly or in part producing the problem, through consultation with a competent physician, and that, if there is such a prior physical condition, proper medical treatment is being administered, and, in such a case, Natural Therapy is being contemplated to deal with the emotional and behavior symptoms that may be persisting.

Beyond that, there are usually some physical symptoms that have originated as a result of one's attitude toward the significant problem that one is experiencing. Such symptoms are often so bizarre and frightening that one can easily find one's self preoccupied only with them, and not with grandiosity.

In addition, some sufferers have read so much about their problem that the origins of their problem have taken on an even more frightening aspect. For example, so much has been written about a so-called subconscious that many appear to believe that they are under the control of some mysterious part of their mind with which they feel helpless to deal, or even to cope. Actually, no one has really proved the existence of such a subconscious. To us, what some describe as a subconscious appears to be nothing more than memory, something that we can all understand and over which exert a great deal of control.

Somewhat akin to this is the theological concept of original sin, to which all ills are often attributed. To view original sin only as an all-pervading tendency to evil, thus possessing some characteristics and effects of the so-called subconcious that we just discussed, is certainly not very helpful in therapy. Certainly, given the history of humankind, it is difficult to deny that there appears to be what someone has aptly described as a basic "cussedness" in everyone. But there has to be some kind of rational and discoverable process, even if one accepts theologically-based considerations, by which such universal "cussedness" can come about. Most logical to us is that it is related to the basic self-interest that everyone has, which insures survival. In that sense, original sin is not so mysterious or even frightening. We are including that idea here, because some with big problems attribute them to past wrongs they have committed and feel that, because of original sin in themselves, they may never be able to be free of their problems.

You can understand, then, how important it is for us to insist that an important prerequisite for implementing Natural Therapy is to fully accept the fact that there is nothing mysterious about the real cause of the problem, because it is grandiosity alone, no matter what symptoms are experienced, or what part any memory of earlier events or even any habitual ways of acting may be playing in the problem.

The *sixth and final prerequisite* is that one must completely avoid the placing of any blame upon one's self or others for one's significant problem. We will not repeat here what we have said earlier about blaming. We refer to blaming here only to indicate that it prevents full and adequate implementation of the therapy. We are aware of the difficulty of avoiding blaming one's self or others for one's plight. Will-power alone will not control it, for it is charged with emotion, and, as it has been said, in any contest between emotion and the will, emotion almost always wins out.

Our advice then is to attempt to outfox it. And this can be done if one reminds one's self that blaming, too, is caused by one's grandiosity. When one blames one's self, one is saying: "A wonderful person like myself should not have done such a thing that has brought about this big problem." When blaming others one is saying: "A great person like myself could not have brought such a bad thing about. I deserve better treatment than that." Thus, whenever tempted to place any blame, it's best to challenge such self-talk with replies like: "No one is really to blame; it's just my grandiosity trying to tell me otherwise."

So much for prerequisites for implementing Natural Therapy. There are others, of course, especially esoteric ones, but we have found that most people have become aware of their special ones by the time they are ready to try a therapy such as this. It might be profitable for everyone to think about any special prerequisites he or she no doubt has, in addition to the general ones we have just described. Such special prerequisites often are suggested by some special habits that have in the past interfered with successfully attempting to carry out a program to solve the problem. No one should overlook the importance of prerequisites, for a neglect of them usually aborts the therapy before it has hardly had a chance to initially prove itself.

IMPLEMENTING THE THERAPY

If you have adequately met the prerequisites we just described you are well on the way to dealing successfully with your significant problem. Our past experiences with those who learned about the therapy, and then took the first steps toward implementing it on the basis of such prerequisites, have furnished us abundant proof that this is true. So, proceed to the payoff by following each step now outlined.

At this point, if you are a religious person, you might want to begin with a prayer. But not just any kind of prayer, and surely not a prayer that is simply a petition that God would assist this therapy to do its work and cure. A proper prayer at this point would be a request for divine help to enable the prayer-er to do what he or she already knows that has to be done. The prayer-er can then proceed on the confident assumption that such assistance will surely be forthcoming.

In our previous book we urged that the first step in the therapy should be to shift the focus to the real problem. There we pointed out that almost always the one with a significant problem is unable to begin solving his problem, because the real problem was obscured by all the symptoms, which themselves became the center of primary attention. As the reader of this book already knows, by requiring the would-be user of the therapy to accept what we say about acquired grandiosity, we have in our updated Natural Therapy already shifted the focus to the real problem.

There is, however, one important consideration in that initial step in the earlier book that has important relevance to the improved procedures we outline here in the present book, and that has to do with the relative amount of calmness and release from tension required to put the various steps of the therapy into actual practice. If that is a present problem for you, as it is likely to be, it can be dealt with even more adequately in the first step we recommend here. So let us go immediately to that.

STEP I. BREAK THE CONTROL OF HAVE-TOS!

By far the best way to overcome tension, even panic, is to take this first step. Those who have heard our AGAPE CASSETTE, designed to control and prevent panic-states, already know that the Natural Therapy method for such control and prevention consists essentially in taking this first step.

To break the control of have-tos it is necessary to become fully convinced that you do not need to discontinue your self-interest. You must rather convince yourself of the legitimacy of your self-interest, and that your self-interest can best be served in the Natural Therapy way. Here's how.

Let's start with your high-tension, even panic states. What in the world does convincing yourself of the legitimacy of your own self-interest have to do with that? The way humans ordinarily view their self-interest is actually the prime cause of tension and panic. They view it in the same terms that we view grandiosity — an almost exclusive interest in serving only one's self. And tension and panic states arise when such self-interest is not being satisfied in interaction with others, when others do not act toward us the way we want them to.

All right, take a good look at your present tensions and even episodes of panic, and you will find that they are being produced somehow in that manner. Look for that phenomenon in your recent or ongoing interaction with other significant or "important" people in your past, present, or future life. You will certainly find it.

You have already admitted your grandiosity when you subscribed to the prerequisites or even before. Now see its effects in your insistence on having others act favorably toward you, and note the outcomes in your tensions and even panic when they don't.

Now recall another prerequisite to which you have subscribed — the Natural Therapy way for overcoming grandiosity, and note how you have not been doing that in your interactions with others. In that way you will realize that trying to serve your self-interest through manipulation of others, or, rather, dependence upon others for feelings about yourself, has brought about your big problems.

So there has been nothing wrong with your interest in yourself, only in the way you tried to go about serving it. You thought you *had to* get them to do for you what you wanted them to do, and that not only failed, but also brought you misery. Now control that have-to, by reminding yourself that *you really don't have to* get your interests served in the ways that you thought you did, or the way your grandiosity impelled you to, but that rather there is another way, a natural way, an easier way, a way that never fails — the Natural Therapy way.

When you have gained sufficient control of your have-tos that you have firmly resolved that you will no longer permit your self-feelings to be at the mercy of what *others* do, but dependent only upon what *you* do, only then are you ready to go on in further implementing the therapy. And you can do so with great confidence, for, if you are to survive and progress, as all of humanity generally has, then there must reside in you and in every other human some means for such survival and progress. Thus the next logical step that you need to take is to search diligently for those means in your own self, as indicated in what now follows.

STEP II. KNOW YOURSELF!

The directions in this section follow the directions we already outlined and rather fully described in chapter two of this book, which, in turn, are based upon the original directions in our previous book. So here we do not dwell any further on the reasons for the various steps and techniques for properly implementing them. Rather we apply them more helpfully on the basis of the insights we have received since the first appearance of the therapy,

A. Know Your Hereditary-Biological Self

As we stated earlier, there is no point in evaluating the environmental influences that have in any way shaped your behavior. The environment simply enabled your biological predispositions to become realities, and also offered the various choices of the form that that reality might take. Important is your inborn degree of conditionability. To repeat, if your significant problem is mainly an emotional one, then you can be quite certain that you are easily-conditioned by outside influences, and were therefore meant to be concerned about human problems. If your significant problems are mainly in the area of behavior or conduct, then you can be quite certain that you are difficult-to-condition by nature, and you were meant to initiate and take action toward the solution of human problems, which your counterparts, the easily-conditioned ones, constantly point out to you.

B. Know That You Are Grandiose

Since you have the kind of conditionability you have, you really are grandiose, or you would not have any significant problem. Look for the grandiosity that is behind your problem, and you will find it. Trace the behavior steps that led to your big problem, and you will eventually see your big ego as the culprit that started it all.

Convince yourself of this again here by analyzing your

have-tos, your compulsions to always act as you do, that finally end up in big problems for you. One of the easiest ways to do this is to really and honestly examine the way you manipulate people for your own purposes. Then see how even this puts you at the mercy of these people, for you must constantly put up the charade, and really you become, in effect, a slave or captive of these people, although it all started out by *your* manipulation of *them.* So you feel trapped and frustrated, and it all becomes quite unbearable, which, in itself, becomes a significant problem, or leads to other, even more significant, problems.

C. Know Your Other Natural Qualities.

While it is your degree of conditionability by external influences that is most important, you have many other inborn qualities that are important in dealing successfully with your problems. The task here is to try to determine the most important ones, the ones that do relate directly to what you were meant to do with your natural qualities. Qualities like degree of intelligence, natural amount of energy, physical characteristics. You already know that you have high emotionality. Make a rather comprehensive and exhaustive list. Ask those who know you well to help. Get professional help in this from those who administer aptitude tests, provide vocational counseling, evaluate health and physical capacities. You will be surprised how bountifully nature has equipped you to perform the job it has laid out for you.

Include in your inventory all the additional abilities and skills you have developed as a result of your natural aptitude for such development, the ones that directly or indirectly can contribute to your carrying out the job that nature has chosen as your most important life's work. Finally, add to the list any additional abilities and skills that you could develop on the basis of your natural aptitudes, and which also relate to your principal mission in life. You may need or want to enlist the help of various kinds of specialists of the kind we mentioned earlier. Seek help from libraries and librarians.

Now you have any number of possibilities for properly and successfully carrying out that mission, and you are becoming enthusiastic and even impatient about pursuing them. Here's how to get started and to carry on with ongoing success.

STEP III. BE YOURSELF!

Of course, we mean only your natural self. Almost everyone knows how counterproductive it is to try to be anyone else. But that is what the grandiose individual has been trying to do. He is trying to live up to an image of himself that does not really exist. So, be your natural self! Here's how.

A. Maximize Yourself

Much of therapy today advocates self-actualization, and by that they usually mean: "Do your own thing." And by that they often mean not only to do what comes naturally to you, but also what you want to do, and finally what you want to do for yourself. With our new look at motivation for the therapy we pretty much go along with that, except to make this most important condition — whatever we find to do in such self-actualization, it must have to do primarily with using ourselves to improve the lot of humankind.

Our direction here is to do two things: 1. improve to the best of your ability those natural qualities that you have, that are related to what you now know is your most important mission in life, and 2. determine present opportunities that exist for you, in the areas of vocation or avocation, to which you can make your maximum contribution. This will take time and effort. Do it.

B. Maximize Yourself Primarily FOR Yourself

Here we are suggesting that you constantly remind yourself that you must practice the therapy as best as you

can for at least two important reasons: 1. your own legitimate self-interest, and 2. the fulfillment of the most important reason why you are who you are.

That kind of constant reminder can only help you to
carry out, whatever you have now found that you must do,
to the best of your ability. All the principles of operant
conditioning and of behavior modification have been carried out most successfully in the control of human
behavior when they have used reward as the ongoing motivating factor. Actually, our former approach to the use of
Natural Therapy, we now see, failed to give adequate
motivation, because it practically used the opposite —
punishment — as the principal motivating factor, although
at the time we did not view it as such.

We formerly were depending on the final reward — the
control of significant problems — to supply sufficient
motivation for tackling the therapy. Apparently that is not
immediate enough, especially for grandiose people. Now
we understand more fully, what almost all therapists com-
plain about, and which we tried to explain and overcome in
the Afterword of our earlier book — the apparent reluctance of so many suffering from some big problems to
plunge headlong into a therapy that, even to them, appears
to offer some important help.

Additionally, we also knew that, once an individual seriously tried to put the therapy into use, however inade-
quately at the beginning, he would soon be receiving initial
favorable feedback to induce him to carry on. In this also
we were erroneous. Oh, the favorable feedback did occur,
even early for most, but it wasn't that great that it could
impart the kind of ongoing motivation we had expected.
We should have known better, because we have often said,
in describing grandiose people, that they want it *all,* and
they want it all *right now!*

Okay, in our new approach, you've got practically all of
it even before you start. When we have used this new approach more recently, we no longer have the initial reac-

tion, at the end of the first counseling session, that we often noted in our former approach. That reaction was sometimes so unenthusiastic, that we sometimes advised clients that they apparently were not ready for the therapy, and that, until they could muster up enough courage and energy to fight their grandiosity in the toe-to-toe and head-on way we apparently were suggesting, they had better not continue in therapy with us.

In the new approach, clients become so enthusiastic that we feel the need to constantly remind them that it's going to take some time, that they can expect setbacks, and the like, before they get in control of their lives again. But it appears that they're not listening. They seem to have the "Eureka!" kind of feeling that characterized the proverbial soldier who walked around picking up paper and muttering to himself: "This isn't it," to the point where they felt they had to discharge him, and, when they handed him his discharge papers, he brightened up and shouted: "This is it!" And that nicely sets the stage for the final direction, which is the heart of the therapy.

C. Maximize Yourself By Maximizing Others

You can do everything else we have suggested up till now, but, if it does not finally culminate in your doing what is directed here, you would only be adding more big problems. Because most of modern therapy actually fails to urge you to go on to what we advise here, it only succeeds in making you feel better, because in their way you are getting your big ego needs satisfied, that big ego that brought your problems to begin with. In addition, in that way the ego is made even bigger, and its demands grow ever larger, producing ever more and bigger problems, and you end up feeling worse than ever.

Only evolution or an omniscient Creator could have designed the paradoxical way, spelled out here, to get individual needs satisfied to the extent that all humanity's needs are satisfied. Now we see ever so clearly that individual self-interest has to exist side by side with altruism, even though we have for so long thought that they were, and had to be, mutually exclusive.

While using your natural qualities to help humankind is the essence of the therapy, we ought to say something more definite about the way you might go about implementing it. We have found that many people seem to find it difficult to know how to do it, especially how to get started. We have mentioned earlier that we have advised some people to start simply by just being friendly to those with whom they interact regularly, like their postman, newsboy, waitress, etc.

We have learned, however, that some take this to mean that helping others is to be typically done in that manner. That suggestion was only to get people to do something to get started, something quite easy to do, and something that provides almost immediate favorable feedback. As an example of the typical kind of therapy, however, it is a very poor one. One could soon get in the habit of doing that just to get one's own ego boosted.

The therapy is to be carried out in a manner in which important and substantial help is given primarily to help others to maximize themselves. In the first place, we have learned the hard way, in the whole area of assisting needy people, that, to give them merely a handout, does them more harm than good. We can help others best by assisting them to maximize *their* lives, even as we are maximizing *ours* by using ourselves primarily to help *them.*

Of course, we may supply some things that they need immediately, just to get into the position where they can learn the need for maximizing themselves; we might have to feed them, improve their health, and in other ways help them with the nuts and bolts of just managing to maintain an adequate existence. We might also assist them to do the things that we ourselves had to do, to learn who we are and to be who we are, as described earlier in this chapter.

This applies to every person whom we are obligated to

help, even if they are severely handicapped, for, no matter what an individual has going for him, or how much, the best way we can assist that individual is to help him make the most of what he is and has, in the same ways that we are doing so ourselves. This may include at times even opposing him, if necessary, if that is the only way to help him to do, what he has to do, to learn how to maximize his own life.

Of course, we first use loving methods, methods that operate on immediate reward. But, when that does not work, we may have to use harsher methods. Sometimes to carry out our own mission to maximize ourselves, or even to help others, if we do not get the cooperation of others involved, through the softer approaches, we may have to use tougher ones. Such considerations involve the dependency relationships we described earlier. Sometimes it may be necessary for us to make them choose between cooperating with us or of ending the relationship. This may sound a little heartless, but, in truth, you are really not helping them by letting such a relationship go on.

Finally, we have found that in attempting to initiate the direction in this section, it is seldom necessary to launch a big search to find the kinds of people you are best equipped to help. Sometimes there are large groups of people who are in need of our help, and we may be able to help them best by helping the social structure, or other environmental condition, to respond more adequately to meet certain needs that certain groups or groupings of people have. The large number of social problems today make it quite unnecessary to make any great search for people that need our help.

Of course, in helping large groups, we must never overlook the prime goal we have of helping individuals to maximize themselves. If any social structure or other environmental situation is functioning to discourage or even prevent the maximizing of individuals, then our help to humankind can best be administered by removing that structure or other environmental situation or by changing its functions, and perhaps an important thing for us to do in such a case is to help individuals affected to understand this, whether they are the people in charge or those that are being victimized.

If you've taken a kind of look around to see the possibilities for you to use yourself for others, and you don't see anything around (this seldom is the case), then just don't tackle any old thing that seems to be at hand. This whole thing doesn't really work that way. The best thing to do is to wait till some opportunity presents itself, and, when it does, you'll really know it, if you've done the preparation we have suggested, and you can go right into action, also with a great deal of know-how and confidence. Until that opportunity comes around, don't just stagnate. Keep on keeping on with maximizing your natural qualities, for something much bigger than you ever imagined may suddenly turn up. We've had many of those experiences ourself.

The emphasis in Natural Therapy is on the natural qualities we have and their employment in the help that they can render to the welfare of humankind. We can certainly endanger the success of the therapy if we give undue emphasis to the individuals whom we seek to help. For one, sometimes the very people we seek to help turn on us, oppose us, criticize us, and may finally not want any part of our help. Such an experience may discourage us from attempting the therapy again.

If we remember that all we are required to do is to render the best help that we can, regardless of who it is that we are led to help, then such adverse reactions do not affect us. In fact, if there is any kind of personal relationship between the helper and the one to be helped, there needs to be an understanding between both parties of the importance of the help itself, above all personal considerations.

Certainly, one cannot go on endlessly without some kind of assurances that it is all worthwhile. Now you see again the importance of our new emphasis on the primacy of our own self-interest in the therapy. If we are doing all this especially in our own interest, we don't need to be affected by any lack of appreciation from others. We have already received our highest reward even before we set out to render our help to others. We have maximized our natural qualities, our real self, not our phony, grandiose self. And we have found our ultimate purpose and mission in life. Knowing that, and being equipped to carry out that mission in the best possible way, who needs others for support, others who, while they may render some support, often let us down, and finally will be lost to us completely by the separation of death?

Practicing the therapy as we suggest it here eliminates such unpleasant outcomes. In fact, it should be a constant source of joy and satisfaction, the like of which you have never known before. To make certain that you don't miss that, our last direction is a reminder, as well as a test, of that.

STEP IV. ENJOY YOURSELF!

Many who practice Natural Therapy have no need for this direction, for they are having the time of their life using it. Some of their statements testify to that, like the following:

> "When I wake up, I immediately wonder what good things are going to happen to me today."

> "Whenever things seem to be going wrong, I've found that there is always something better coming up."

> "For the first time in my life, I don't care what others think of what I do or say."

> "I've never had so much to do, and I never enjoyed so much doing it."

But we are including this reminder, because some apparently have been in the clutch of their grandiosity and have-tos so long, they are almost afraid to enjoy themselves.

It is not unusual, when someone has achieved some control of his grandiosity and his problem with it, that we are asked: "What do I do now?" or, "Where are all those goodies I'm supposed to get?" And all that we have to do is to tell them to look around, and we give a few examples of the many great rewards that are there just for the taking. Like: "Now you can take that job you always wanted to have, but were afraid to tackle before," or, "Now quit letting people use you for their own selfish purposes," or, "Your first duty is toward fulfilling your prime purpose in life; and everything and everybody else can best be served, if you do not permit them to interfere with that."

Their favorable reaction to that is fast and often furious, so much so that sometimes we found ourselves having to advise them to slow down and not overdo it. It is rather thrilling to hear about the kinds of exhilaration so many apparently are experiencing, once they have Natural Therapy going for them. We sometimes find it hard to believe the results some people are apparently achieving.

So, if you are trying to practice the therapy in earnest for any length of time, and are not finding yourself enjoying it, perhaps you are not using it right. And we can only advise that you read over carefully what we have written in this book — all of it — and then try again. It's just got to work. It's scientifically true, and it's natural law, so the great Dr. Hans Selye testifies.

If you're a religious person, we know of no religion that does not promise divine blessings upon our using ourselves to help others. Biblical Christians have this promise: "The blessing of the Lord, it maketh rich, and he addeth *no sorrow with it.*"

When's the last time you really had a good time? Without artificial stimulants, we mean. If you're grandiose, you might have a hard time remembering. Well, Natural Therapy offers another chance to enjoy yourself again, even while you use it.

chapter **8**

*Some Typical
Applications*

APPLICATIONS ALWAYS BASICALLY THE SAME

While already in the third chapter we have given some
glimpses into the application of the therapy to common
significant problems, in this concluding chapter we try to
indicate how the therapy may be applied to practically all
problem areas. Of course, this is a large territory to cover,
so we have had to limit this description mostly to general
problem areas, rather than to the more specific ones. Even
then, some may still regard this venture as overly-
ambitious, but, because Natural Therapy is designed for
significant problems, and holds that for them there is only
one basic cause, and therefore need only one basic cure,
we feel that our task is not that difficult.

We would readily agree that, for minor problems, an
individual can be helped even if he only can tell his problems to someone else, or if someone else will just sit and
listen and understand and sympathize, and then end up
saying simply: "Someday this, too, shall pass." And it
usually does.

But significant emotional and behavior problems are always the result of grandiosity and ensuing have-tos, and it is always the control of grandiosity that finally also controls the significant problem. Even if the problem is one like ill-health. When we were discovering, to our great amazement, the utility of Natural Therapy for just about any problem, we finally came to the problem of severe physical pain. Could the therapy be helpful even for that?

As a parish pastor we had served many individuals who had that problem, especially in cases of incurable cancer. Very often, while such individuals were just languishing at home, awaiting the arrival of the grim reaper, we often found them lying in their beds as miserable as anyone could ever be. Sometimes their busy physicians never took time to tell them what they might do at home to lessen some of that misery. Sometimes they were in nursing homes, and the nurse in charge would ask us to help such individuals get into a better frame of mind, for so many had given up, so many were always complaining, and, in general, they were making themselves more miserable by their attitudes.

We tried to distract them from their preoccupation with their sad plight. If they were ambulatory we'd ask: "What are you doing there in bed all the time?" They'd often answer: "Don't you know I'm dying?" We'd answer: "If I were you, I'd want to die with my boots on." That usually didn't help for too long, for the next time we visited them we'd have to cajole them into getting out of bed again and doing something. We had a little better success when we advised those sufferers, either ambulatory or bedfast, to use themselves to help others, even if it was possible only to pray for them — another example of our earlier intuitions that helped lead us to Natural Therapy.

Of course, a few became angry at our suggestions, which often appeared to some as quite unsympathetic, but even that gave them something other than their misery to think about. These earlier experiences with the problem of severe pain, together with our ongoing discovery of the widespread utility of our therapy, led us to research the pain problem further. It brought us into contact with persons like Dr. Ronald Katz of UCLA, head of its anesthesiology department and director of its two pain clinics. Through his work we learned how such pain could be managed, even when the usual treatments through medication and surgery could not provide adequate relief, often through psychological approaches.

Earlier we had learned a great deal about such an approach through our close association with Dr. Barbara B. Brown, foremost authority on biofeedback. For a while we worked together to try to establish an early biofeedback center in the Los Angeles area. Through such associations it was easy to see how our Natural Therapy could make a contribution.

Essentially that which makes any situation a problem, for those involved in it, is not the situation itself, but the attitude of the individuals toward it. It's quite evident that grandiose individuals cannot often accept a problem situation that apparently cannot be changed, also in the case of illness or injury accompanied by great pain. But our therapy can modify that grandiosity enough to bring a certain amount of relief, either by reducing the tensions that may be adding to it, or by lessening the accompanying mental and emotional anguish, usually inevitable in pain and adding to the misery, or by both.

Incidentally, in our experience with biofeedback, we learned that some individuals find it difficult to relax enough to achieve the so-called "alpha state," or to stay in it for any length of time. We can now see how, through our therapy, an individual's tension could be so reduced as to make this important requisite for using biofeedback much easier to meet.

What we have thus far stated in this introductory section has taken us into the body of the chapter, for we have given a sample of the therapy's application even to problems that are usually not regarded as essentially emotional or behavioral, problems like poverty and ill-health, which certainly are significant ones for a large segment of the population.

To make this first sample of the use of the therapy for this general area complete, we need to add some important information about significant problems, which are as significant as they are, because they are due to a combination of biological causes supplemented by grandiosity. An example here is chronic depression. It is commonly accepted today that there are various kinds of depression, usually distinguished on the basis of their origin.

While psychotherapy in general has not been as helpful for ongoing depression as it often proclaims, it has been our discovery that this is often due to the over-simplistic approach commonly made. Often the biological factor is completely overlooked. Natural Therapy on the other hand, has had some of its greatest success with the kind of depression that is often the most difficult to overcome — the kind that is the result of a biological predisposition plus grandiosity.

While the biological element that evidently produces the predisposition is not adequately clear at this time, it certainly is very helpful in therapy to recognize the strong evidence for the existence of such a biological predisposition, which is usually apparent when the kinds of life adjustments of parents and siblings are ascertained.

We have found, in treating depressives who have not been helped by other therapists, because neither the grandiosity nor the biological aspects have been recognized or treated, that helping the client to understand and accept the biological aspects, that are often present, is necessary to bring adequate relief. The nice thing about this is that, to accomplish both the reduction of grandiosity and the acceptance of the biological predisposition, the same therapy is employed.

We are thus led to make this general observation that has a great deal of utility, especially where grandiosity has been significantly reduced, but some symptomatology persists: in such instances, for lack of any better information, the client ought to accept the likely possibility of a biological predisposition being involved, and, through ongoing control of grandiosity, continue to accept this and live with it, as long as the biological element, or whatever else might be discovered as playing a part, is not adequately controlled. The knowledge that one is emoting or behaving essentially, or to a large exent, because of some such biological predisposition, we have found, serves to prepare an individual for such an eventuality, and thus forearm him or her often to blunt its initial impact, as well as to employ the mechanisms of control, suggested by our therapy, with a great deal of calm and confidence.

What we have just stated holds true, at least in our present state of knowledge, even for problems, where we have not yet discovered any such biological predisposition, but where some symptomatology persists despite an apparently adequate control of grandiosity.

Incidentally, it is our prediction that a biological basis, of the kind that we've just been describing, will increasingly be found to be playing a part in certain types of significant emotional and behavior problems. At the same time, the increasing isolation of the actual physical mechanism involved, which we also envision, will certainly hasten also their adequate control. We feel the Natural Therapy makes some contribution toward that eventuality.

Before going on to other general areas to which the therapy can be applied, we ought to say something about the use of medication for significant problems. In problems where there is apparently some physical cause contributing to the problem, such medication may be helpful, but should be prescribed only to the degree that it is necessary to help the client gain enough control to better utilize Natural Therapy. While in all cases, we always advise that the final decision regarding medication should be made by competent medical practitioners, those taking such medication should be aware of two important aspects that may be involved.

It commonly occurs that those, who are using the therapy and are at the same time taking prescribed medication, have actually gained such control of their grandiosity that they really have no need for the medication any longer, or at least in the amounts that they needed it up till then. However, they may have also become physically attuned to it enough to experience enough withdrawal symptoms to make them concerned about whether they really are coming into control of their problem. Such concerns often can resurrect some ghosts of grandiosity from which they had thought they had freed themselves.

What we have done in such situations, when we have assured ourselves that grandiosity had really been significantly controlled, has been to try to explain to the clients the facts of the situation, and to suggest that they approach their medical adviser about the possibility of modifying the medication. It is not unusual, when such modification has been made, that there soon comes a day when the client begins to forget to take his medication, although we always advise that they tell their physician about this before they discontinue it completely on their own.

It should be added that there are no doubt some, who have physical involvements of such a degree, that they may have to continue to take medication on an ongoing basis, just as some individuals have such malfunction of their insulin-producing organs that they need to take ongoing medication for their diabetic symptoms. The control of grandiosity can help individuals accept also that prospect with equanimity.

While we stated already in our earlier book that, when those, whose problems are only of functional origin, without a physical cause, are so upset that they are not able to put the therapy into practice, some sedation may be indicated, it should not be excessive or prolonged. While even excessive and prolonged sedation and other medication may have occurred, the therapy can still be used, but it may take a little longer to implement it as effectively as it could be under ordinary circumstances. At the same time, as we have also tried to make clear in everything we have stated here about medication, one can look forward to eventually gaining some control despite that tougher beginning.

PREVENTION OF SIGNIFICANT PROBLEMS

While Natural Therapy came out originally as a treatment, its most important contribution has to be its use for the avoidance of such problems, for prophylaxis. We often meet up with environmental-determinists who argue that, even if biological determinism were true, we have only the environment to use for therapy.

This, of course, is not true either. However, so as not to waste time in fruitless argument with such an objection, that betrays a great deal of ignorance about biological determinism and how it is operative in human behavior, we simply indicate the therapy's important significance for the *prevention* of significant problems. Over against that there can be no effective argument, for the environmental determinists have had their day for using the environment to prevent important problems, and the results have been not only unproductive, but actually and tragically counterproductive. Important problems, personal and social, are increasing by leaps and bounds.

In all that follows in this chapter, we try to show how the Natural Therapy approach is highly useful in both the prevention and the amelioration of significant problems. We feel certain that readers are sufficiently acquainted with our therapy to make all the proper applications of the principles of the therapy, either for prevention or for solution, to all the areas treated in the remainder of this chapter, so that we need not continually spell it out.

INTERPERSONAL RELATIONSHIPS, IN GENERAL

Since we have repeatedly stated that all significant problems are problems in interpersonal relationships of one sort or another, some personal, others impersonal, we make several statements here that are generally relevant to all the specific areas that we treat in all that follows. While counselors these days so often lay the blame for problems in this area to lack of communication, and often hold out to their clients the magic cure of "communication," we have so often been approached by many of these same clients for help, because the communication approach has not worked for them.

That's understandable, for, unless one knows where the other person is coming from, on the basis of degree of conditionability and grandiosity, and, unless one also knows where one is coming from one's self in both these areas, one does not know what to communicate, or how to communicate properly to begin with. In fact, it is only on the basis of such knowledge that one can understand the reason for lack of communication in the first place. What we've just pointed out here is the most important basic consideration in any concern about causes of problems or their cure.

Of lesser importance, but still important are the following, which also have an intimate relationship with what we've just stated, but which need to be explained further, mostly because of the vast amount of misinformation being peddled about them. First there is the issue of *the need to be loved.* In general, we are in agreement with Albert Ellis when he states that we do not need to be loved; we have only been taught that we need love. The only exceptions we would make would be the showing of unconditional love to infants not yet in conscious control of their behavior, and, as Glasser also suggests in his Reality Therapy, to others whom we are trying to help overcome a significant problem. In the latter, we would use it as a means of motivating the individual to accept our help. As soon as he might view it as a weakness on our part, and use it to excuse his actions, we might very well modify that love considerably. It is understood, of course, that by the term "love," we mean affection, liking, acceptance, etc., and not especially the *agape* we spoke about in chapter three, which portrays the ongoing feelings of concern which we need to have for all humankind.

We would also agree with those who hold that there is generally a much greater danger in giving too much love than in giving too little. It must be remembered that, when one has true self esteem, which can only be acquired by using one's self in the ways we indicate in our therapy, one does not need the love of another for the acquiring or maintenance of one's self-image, as we've explained earlier. Anyway, such adequate self-images cannot be imposed from without, by others, by therapists, or even by the individual himself through his own positive thinking about himself, and the like. It only comes naturally, when the individual earns for himself that self-esteem by acting in accordance with the design for his life.

Hate, of the kind that makes for significant problems in interpersonal relationships, is a result of the have-tos, acquired from grandiosity, that augment the high emotionality of those at the extremes of conditionability. Extreme *anger* and *hostility,* as well as *envy* and *jealousy* stem from the same sources.

Many of the most significant problems in this area are found among *relatives.* Much of this is due to what we have already stated, that relatives have become very dependent upon each other as insurers of their own self-esteem and self-image. Because of the great misunderstanding about the need for being loved, and being loved unconditionally, that is found especially among relatives, interpersonal problems among such individuals are some of the most painful, because so much is at stake, as we've just pointed out.

We've earlier demonstrated that the dependencies involved may have to be modified, or even eliminated, if the problems are to be solved, but only non-grandiose individuals can do so with equanimity. It's not just enough to recognize that, if one is a relative of another, it is, except for the marriage partner, an accidental relationship, over which one has no choice, although it makes the severing of dependencies easier.

PARENTHOOD AND CHILD-REARING

While it is true that prevention of significant problems must begin as soon as a child is born (a good case can be made for starting it even *in utero,* but we will not treat this, except as it relates to what we say about mate-selection), much earlier preparation for it must be made for it already when planning for marriage, or for living together, that eventuates in possible child-bearing.

In preparing for marriage, of course, the welfare of one spouse is associated most importantly with the welfare of the mate, and compatibility, which is generally accepted as the most important element for a successful marriage, only is maximized as the partners maximize themselves and their mates in ways that Natural Therapy suggested in the previous chapter. Naturally, due consideration must be given to the degrees of conditionability and the have-tos possessed by each partner, if one is to select the proper future mate with whom such compatibility can be effected.

If plans for marriage include also offspring, then that necessitates a great deal of insight from Natural Therapy principles, if that is to be done for the best interests of everyone concerned, which actually includes all of humanity. Again special attention needs to be paid to what type of inborn degree of conditionability the child or children are likely to inherit.

And, after the child is born, one needs to know rather precisely its degree of conditionability so as to avoid grandiosity. Of course, it is obvious that one ought to try to determine that as early as possible, and that is not always easy at the beginning, with the knowledge we have at present. The avoidance of grandiosity, and even proper socialization, necessitate doing the same things that are involved in solving significant problems, helping the child to maximize himself by maximizing himself for the maximizing of others. With so many parents, terrified of warping their child's personality, actually helping to do so by an overabundance of unconditional love (except when they do so in the exceptional cases we mentioned in the previous section), it is vitally important that they help the child develop true self-esteem and self-confidence, in the ways we have suggested.

FORMAL EDUCATION

Children, while basically set in the ways they tend to act spontaneously by the time they leave the home for formal schooling outside the home, are still pliable enough to be influenced in some degree by school experiences. Parents and school authorities ought to be fully aware of the importance of the principles of human behavior that are involved with Natural Therapy, if they seek to be successful in the educational process. Only that kind of approach can assure proper motivation for teaching and learning.

The constantly changing and differing methodologies, so characteristic of American education, is an indication to us that education really does not seem to know where the pupil is coming from. If it were known, there could be only one basic method of educating that pupil. But because of the inborn differences in pupils, which education apparently does not yet adequately appreciate, it often seems that the methodology is not working as well as could be expected, when applied to an entire class.

Any good teacher knows that the mere outpouring of all the knowledge, he desires to impart in a particular academic area, does not guarantee that the pupil will make proper use of it. As the old saying has it, it isn't what you know that counts, but how you feel about it. Unless he knows where an individual is coming from, in terms of his kind of conditionability and his kind of have-tos, if any, no teacher can properly meet a student's needs and interests, which are the prime determiners of how he is going to feel about any information.

MARRIAGE AND FAMILY PROBLEMS

Just about every important problem that arises in this area has been already treated in whatever we have said in this book about interpersonal relationships and child-rearing.

SEX PROBLEMS

In addition to the obvious importance again of basic conditionability and have-tos in sex problems, another natural consideration is the basic difference in the sexual nature of the male and the female. Environmental determinists have tried to obscure some important differences here, such as the male drive being associated more importantly with physical tensions, but the female drive being more diffuse and not initially associated with such an ongoing tension, but rather with an induced tension, and, more importantly with the need for assurances of love, regard, faithfulness, and the like.

But the basic problem involved in difficulties associated with sex does not have to do with ignorance, or even with psychological upsets that may cause functional frigidity and impotence. Certainly, they do cause problems, but the problems assume significance only where there is grandiosity, and subsequent have-tos, involved. If one examines the rather successful techniques that therapists like Masters and Johnson employ for sex problems, it is quite evident that the mere willingness alone of subjecting one's self to the techniques involves an initial control of have-tos, also as a result of the greater good that the individual expects to finally receive, as well as the control of grandiosity involved in learning to maximize one's self by maximizing others, which is also involved in the procedure, could easily be the keys to the success of such therapy.

One could not very well condemn masturbation, *per se,* on Natural Therapy grounds, but certainly excessive masturbation (to the point where it is performed when not really needed) could be classified as another have-to that one could learn to control, through the control of grandiosity.

An application of the therapy to premarital and extramarital sex, which are considered a problem by many and to many, is beyond the scope of our intentions for this chapter. If anyone could give us an adequate definition of what the essence of marriage is, we might attempt it.

We do not feel that homosexuality is essentially any greater problem than heterosexuality, for in each instance there are restrictions regarding its free exercise. Our feeling is that it is a have-to to insist on complete freedom in these areas. It is, finally, the part that our need, to use ourselves primarily for the survival and progress of humankind, plays in these areas that should determine any license for, or limitation to, our desired behavior in these kinds of activities.

ADDICTIVE-TYPE BEHAVIOR

Common problems in this area are alcoholism, narcotic drug addiction, and compulsive gambling. These are sometimes called victimless crimes, but there are always at least two victims — the individual indulging in them and the members of society that have to pay for their rehabilitation and for the support of their dependents. Addicts are essentially of two types: the ones that indulge mainly for some kind of emotional support (the easily-conditioned ones), and the ones that indulge mainly for kicks (the difficult-to-condition ones). All of them, of course, have important have-tos.

ECONOMIC PROBLEMS

Some of the things mentioned in connection with our reference to problems of ill-health apply equally here, especially when any economic problem is not due to any fault of the one having it. Thus those with such problems as poverty and unemployment, through no fault of their own, might note what we state about the use of our therapy for ill-health, and find some applications that may be indicated. Beyond this, of course, if economic problems are due to any functional laziness, or a similar failure to do one's part, then the problem is due mainly to have-tos, and the therapy for grandiosity needs to be applied.

If the problems are due to the structure or function of the structure involved, then the therapy principles need to be applied to, or by, or both, those who control the structure and/or its functions, to make them more responsive to the needs of all involved. This is an instance in which one can see the ways in which each type of basic conditionability can play a part in helping to make the necessary changes. The same principle is applicable to all employer-employee relationship problems, as well as to citizen-government relationship problems, which are mounting alarmingly these days, also because of the increasing bureaucratization of both industry and government.

ALL OF LIFE'S STAGES

Each major life-stage has its particular and special problems, and we treat here only the major ones. We've already considered problems related to childhood, so we begin here with *adolescence,* a particularly stormy period of life. It is generally agreed that, probably as a result of the hormonal changes that occur in the body, adolescents develop an adolescent egocentricity, a phenomenon with which probably all of us are familiar. If they already are grandiose before reaching this stage, then certainly it is easy to understand our contention that, while all adolescents have some problems during this period (the easily-conditioned battle shyness, sensitivity, etc., while the difficult-to-condition indulge in a great deal of clowning and self-display), it is only the grandiose ones that have the big problems (like the easily-conditioned ones feeling greatly inferior, and the difficult-to-condition ones becoming delinquents), problems that hang on long after adolescent egocentricity has waned.

This stage is followed by *young adulthood* whose special problems have to do with identity and finding the answers to: Who am I? and, What am I supposed to do with my life? It would appear that the two major directions in the therapy itself are tailor-made for this age-group: Know yourself! and, Be yourself!

Middle-age is a stage where many pause to look back to see what they have done, and look forward and see that time is running out. Of course, the non-grandiose are able to enjoy whatever the past has brought to them, even if only memories. The grandiose are upset, for it's still possible to make those great dreams come true, and they try to go into higher gear, though with less energy and with even less confidence. Again, it's grandiosity and have-tos that make the difference in outlook. We're not judging which outlook is better, but which will have the bigger problems. Perhaps the latter outlook might benefit humankind more, if grandiosity could be modified. Then again, that kind probably could not succeed without the more patient, relaxed, plodding, and powerful-by-sheer-virtue-of-their-great-number support of the other kind (the moderately-conditionable).

Old age is for so many these days a return to a stage of dependency on others. Certainly a dependency based upon the need for fulfillment of physical needs is an important one for many. Even if such dependency is due to something beyond their control, some are highly upset by it — the grandiose ones, of course. When some, even though not as physically or economically dependent as those we just described, are still dependent upon others for the maintenance of their self-esteem, they have an even greater problem. They often are the grouches, the chronic complainers, the dissatisfied-with-everything crowd. Their have-tos have them still in their control. But, even from that, they can extricate themselves, and conclude also this final stage of earthly life graciously, as we have seen a good number of them do.

THE BOTTOM LINE

With this chapter of brief examples of the application of Natural Therapy to wide and general areas of living, we conclude this book. If you have big problems and have read with understanding what we have written here, then you may now be expecting some concluding inspirational sentence, some encouraging word, or some fiery challenge to fight the adversary with the newly-discovered weapons described in this book. We really have none, nor do you need any. The therapy doesn't operate that way.

It is rather the relaxed but steady, hour-by-hour, day-by-day, week-by-week, month-by-month, and, in some cases, even year-by-year, ongoing, lifting-yourself-up-and-trying-again-after-stumbling-or-falling, little-by-little, inch-by-inch putting its principles into action, wherever there is a possibility to do so, that brings its blessed results.

The bottom line is: *Do it!*

When you do, you'll stop whining and start winning.

acknowledgements . . .

The use of the pronoun "we," and derivatives, throughout this book is not merely the editorial we, but our way of trying to acknowledge that a number of people gave invaluable assistance to the development of Natural Therapy to its present state, and, although the author himself takes sole responsibility for the contents of this book, he desires here to express his gratitude to the many individuals who were very helpful: . . . behavioral scientists Hans Selye, Hans Eysenck, Camilla Anderson, and Albert Ellis for ongoing interest and direct assistance . . . psychologist Frederick Kramer for help in test-construction and computer work . . .our students in recent years for help in test-construction and data gathering, especially Judy Ehlen and Paula Meyer; Kris Walcott especially for acting as recorder and announcer for our radio programs; Karla Braafladt most notably for help in composing radio scripts and for performing as interviewer and sometimes interviewee for all of them . . . avid student of the therapy and promoter of it in the Midwest Sylvia Monson . . . earlier classmate and fellow-pastor Ken Zank, who has lent ongoing encouragement through his interest, and given the therapy exposure on radio and in the press in the Northwest . . . all those we are privileged to counsel with the therapy and who are a constant inspiration to us . . . above all, our good wife Dorothy for her continued loyalty, support, and assistance in every way . . . our son Michael who is also supportive and very helpful in letting us use him as a sounding board for new ideas . . . our daughter Madeleine French who has been helpful also through her typing work.

A few days ago a very fine young lady, whom it was once our great pleasure to counsel, phoned us to say: "I thank God for you. You have been the answer to my prayers." We can conclude these acknowledgements in a no more appropriate way than to pass her sentiments on to all of those we have mentioned above, who are more deserving of them than we are, and to whom, in conclusion, I would like to say the same.

h.m.

SOME ADDITIONAL HELPFUL
SUGGESTED READING

Anderson, Camilla M. "The Pot and the Kettle." in O. Hobart Mowrer's *Morality and Mental Health.* Chicago: Rand McNally and Company, 1967, pp. 196-202. An address to a pastoral conference in which the author describes grandiosity, also as it affects pastors and psychiatrists.

Anderson, Camilla M. "Guilt Is Not The Problem," in *The Pastoral Counselor,* Fall, 1964. A fine presentation showing why grandiosity is the real problem and not guilt which therapists are always trying to treat.

Anderson, Camilla M. "The Self-Image: A Theory of the Dynamics of Behavior, Updated," in *Mental Hygiene,* 55 (July, 1971), pp. 365-368. An outline of this psychiatrist's progress in developing her theory of behavior; shows where grandiosity fits in.

Ansbacher, Heinz L. and Ansbacher, Rowena R. *The Individual Psychology of Alfred Adler.* New York: Harper and Row, 1956. A fine presentation of Adler's basic psychology by which one can see its high relevancy to Natural Therapy.

Ansbacher, Heinz L. and Ansbacher, Rowena R. *Superiority and Social Interest.* Evanston: Northwestern University Press, 1970. Another summary of the two important aspects of Adler's psychology that are also important in Natural Therapy.

Ellis, Albert and Harper, Robert A. *A New Guide to Rational Living.* Englewood Cliffs, N.J.: Prentice-Hall, Inc., 1975. A fine example of the practical use of Rational-Emotive Therapy, which has many features found in Natural Therapy.

Eysenck, Hans J. *The Biological Basis of Personality.* Springfield, Ill.: Charles C. Thomas, 1967. A helpful book to understand biological aspects of human behavior.

Eysenck, Hans J. *Crime and Personality*. London: Routledge and Kegan Paul, 1977. This is the revised edition of the book that turned us on.

Eysenck, Hans J. *Eysenck On Extraversion*. New York: John Wiley and Sons, 1973. Contains Eysenck's more important findings on extraversion-introversion.

Eysenck, Hans J. *Fact and Fiction in Psychology*. Baltimore: Penguin Books, 1965. Shows how psychology can discover important truths by using proper methodology. Undergirds much in Natural Therapy.

Ensenck, Hans J. and Wilson, G. D. *A Textbook of Human Psychology*. Baltimore: University Park Press, 1976. A fine textbook for an introduction to psychology for those who have never had one, and a fine book to help those, who have had the typical American exposure, to obtain more empirical information.

Fosdick, Harry Emerson. *On Being A Real Person*. New York: Harper and Row, 1943. An early classic on therapy from a religious point of view. Chapter IV especially shows a fine grasp of grandiosity.

Journal of Individual Psychology. The semi-annual journal of the North American Society of Adlerian Psychology, Inc. Helpful to update Adler-type thinking and practice.

Maleske, Herald. *Natural Therapy*. Reseda, CA: Mojave Books, 1976. Our first attempt to put Natural Therapy together. Gives some additional background material and also programs of cognitive behavior modification not spelled out in the new book.

Selye, Hans. *Stress Without Distress*. Philadelphia: J. B. Lippincott Co., 1974. In our opinion a book which treats important ingredients of a viable therapy for human problems as Natural Therapy does, but especially from a scientific point of view throughout by a scientist who is the foremost authority on stress.